Dearest Wal[...]

It is my supreme pleasure to place this book in your hands. I hope it inspires you to never look at the feet the same way again.

May the feet be with you ♡

Sam

FOOT READING

A Reflexology Primer
on Foot Assessment

Sam Belyea

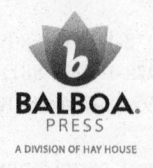

BALBOA PRESS
A DIVISION OF HAY HOUSE

Copyright © 2017 Sam Belyea.

All rights reserved. No part of this book may be used or reproduced by any means, graphic, electronic, or mechanical, including photocopying, recording, taping or by any information storage retrieval system without the written permission of the author except in the case of brief quotations embodied in critical articles and reviews.

This book is a work of non-fiction. Unless otherwise noted, the author and the publisher make no explicit guarantees as to the accuracy of the information contained in this book and in some cases, names of people and places have been altered to protect their privacy.

Balboa Press books may be ordered through booksellers or by contacting:

Balboa Press
A Division of Hay House
1663 Liberty Drive
Bloomington, IN 47403
www.balboapress.com
1 (877) 407-4847

Because of the dynamic nature of the Internet, any web addresses or links contained in this book may have changed since publication and may no longer be valid. The views expressed in this work are solely those of the author and do not necessarily reflect the views of the publisher, and the publisher hereby disclaims any responsibility for them.

The author of this book does not dispense medical advice or prescribe the use of any technique as a form of treatment for physical, emotional, or medical problems without the advice of a physician, either directly or indirectly. The intent of the author is only to offer information of a general nature to help you in your quest for emotional and spiritual well-being. In the event you use any of the information in this book for yourself, which is your constitutional right, the author and the publisher assume no responsibility for your actions.

Any people depicted in stock imagery provided by Thinkstock are models, and such images are being used for illustrative purposes only.
Certain stock imagery © Thinkstock.

Print information available on the last page.

ISBN: 978-1-5043-8809-2 (sc)
ISBN: 978-1-5043-8811-5 (hc)
ISBN: 978-1-5043-8810-8 (e)

Library of Congress Control Number: 2017914395

Balboa Press rev. date: 09/20/2017

Acknowledgements

To understand that anything you create is not your possession alone is the purpose of this section. My unique brand of luck has placed specific people in my life to hone, refine and encourage those attributes in myself that I didn't even know existed. The most influential of those has been my partner Richard. There is nothing that I could say to describe the yoking he has gifted to me through his influence, love and admiration – Thank You.

Surrounding Richard and I's relationship, there have been a series of close encounters that could only be described as formative. Those include my work with teachers like Jennifer Leavy and Sarasvati Devi of what is now Pose by Pose Yoga, who gave me the forum to find my speaking voice as a teacher and who let me leave when it was my time to start my Reflexology training program. Bob Linde and Renee Crozier Prince of Traditions School of Herbal Studies also enthusiastically dusted off my ability and confidence to assess based on elemental theory. Likewise, Christopher Penczak, whose time-tested traditions have continued to push my limits in spiritual practice.

There are many others who I cannot hope to name in this work that have stood by my side and they know who they are. However, I would like to extend special thanks to the people who discouraged me along the way, who did not see my vision and who fought against my framework, only to make it stronger. Many allies have supported me along this journey, but equally so I have been torn down; throughout all of this, I have become who I am today with this book as testament to the fruits of my trials.

Finally, it is to you dear reader that I would like to extend my thanks. Without you picking up this book, the information in these pages could not pass from me to you and thank you for your efforts, curiosity and persistence. It's you that I wrote this book for, the next generation of Foot Reading enthusiasts who will follow me, continue to validate this work and take it to new heights. Use this book in good health and hopefully one day you will be writing an acknowledgement page for your own and will be able to thank your readers in the same fashion.

Sincerely,

Sam Belyea

Contents

Introduction ix

Mapping the Feet 1
    The Origins of Reflexology 3
    How we Map the Feet Physically 4
    The Mental/Emotional Meaning of the Zones 12
    Vertical Zones of Influence 15
    Additional Nuances when Mapping the Feet 19

Elements of a Symptom 23
    Earth 24
    Common Earth Symptomology by Zone 25
    Air 36
    Common Air Symptomology by Zone 37
    Fire 48
    Common Fire Symptomology by Zone 49
    Water 59
    Common Water Symptomology by Zone 60
    Blended Elements 69

Coaching Through the Feet 71
    Putting it all Together 72
    Using the Right Adjectives and Key Words 74
    Ethical Considerations 82
    Methods of Balancing the Elements 85
    Sample Client Scenarios 89

Documenting your Foot Reading Consultations 91
Generating a Foot Reading Report 100

Exploring the Other Extremities 105
Mapping the Hands 106
Mapping the Face 114
Mapping the Ears 123

The Story Continues with You 133

Introduction

On a daily basis I explore the hidden world of feet; decoding the messages held within our five-toed friends and relaying that information to their owners in an effort to heal the bond between the individual and their body. It is with great pleasure that I sit down to write this book because discovering this content was life changing for me, as I hope it will be for you. There is a magic that is present when you are able to see into an individual and understand their makeup, but it is another thing entirely to demonstrate the physical validation that solidifies that intuitive understanding; foot reading has done that for me and can for you. The applications for this knowledge are limited only by the imagination. Before we begin that process of imagining, let's outline the content you are about to pour yourself over.

This book contains the compilation of my understandings about the body and how the body's interconnected nature is entirety represented, in full, on the extremities – specifically the feet. However, I am not just referring to the physical. Another truth I have validated through my foot work is that the body is linked to the internal mental and emotional states of an individual. Not in a pie-in-the-sky, tree-hugging, kumbaya way, but a concretely map-able and observable way. Our state is made manifest through the various bone, muscle, and fluid pathways via the power of our nervous system, which uses both our physical and internal blueprint simultaneously. These two premises, that the whole of the body is mirrored on the individual part and that the mental/emotional state is intertwined with the physical form, are the basis of my work.

Likewise, this content is alive. I cannot accurately explain how it is alive, but I feel as though I have been guided through every step of this journey by the feet themselves. The idea of reading the interconnectedness present within the tissues of our bodies through the feet has a massive gravitational pull over my being and because of that I believe that this work desires to grow through being shared. I will allow the experts of creativity, such as Elizabeth Gilbert in her book *Big Magic*, to further explain the fullest extent of being partnered with such a blazing ball of creative thought-form. That is to say, I am also learning more and more every day about the volumes of information contained within the visual and textural patterns of the feet themselves. I am sure I will reprint these concepts many times in the future as I expand my awareness of the subject, but at this time allow me to share with you what I have come to understand.

This book is arranged to gradually build your knowledge of core foot reading concepts. First, we will begin by explaining the zones and their significance to mapping physical, mental and emotional sections onto the feet. Next, we will discuss symptomology in depth through the theory of four elements: Earth, Air, Fire and Water to describe the various distortions and their meaning that you will come across when assessing the tissues of the feet. Once a mapping framework and vocabulary are built, we will dive into the art of assessment and putting together the story that the feet are trying to tell. Finally, I will expand into the other three extremities and allow those more passionately drawn to reading the hands, face and ears to explore that additional content after the foot reading fundamentals have been understood.

Take the following information in slowly, like a good tea. Sip it and enjoy it. Let the principals and definitions roll around your mental taste buds until the overarching themes are fully known and integrated. I have included many stories within this text about my personal experiences within my Reflexology practice to better explain the various concepts in depth. Likewise, you will find that cross-referencing this work with your previous foot experiences, and those of friends/family, will be very validating and enlightening about the true interconnectedness that has been present this entire time right under your nose – or, rather, under your feet.

As with all true practices, the art comes after the science. Mastering the basics takes time and repetition, looking and feeling many feet is essential. This collection of information is meant to be a starting block for that process. Everything is wonderful in theory and on paper, but living this practice in the real world is what will produce excellence. For now, enjoy the ideas and concepts within these pages, but know that to get good at the art and science of foot reading requires constant reinforcement of the basic principles. No one can do the pushups for you, so get out and see some feet!

Mapping the Feet

Reflexology is where this entire journey started for me. I didn't intend to work with feet; I didn't even consider it an option until I had hit a personal wall in my bodywork practice back in 2010. I was working too hard and blew out my shoulder. I subsequently threw myself into workshops on massage technique and tried to learn how to work smarter to save my body and better serve my clients. Exploring other manual therapies, I realized that they were mostly, with a few quality exceptions, trying to force their will onto the tissues of the body. I knew that the body's pain was a message that begged to be listened to, not simply hammered on until it relented. I needed to find a practice that listened and addressed the body's call for help and that spark of a desire dragged me into my first Reflexology class against my will.

The flyer for that fateful Reflexology class, I had actually thrown in the trash. Seriously, that's what happened. It was my partner Richard who literally reached into the trash, pulled the flyer back out, handed it back to me and said the magic words of, "Try it. You might like it." At the time, I didn't expect to find everything I was searching for within the feet, but I did end up going to that class. The experience taking the course was average, nothing special, but the practical side of the work is what blew me away. Taking the foot techniques back to the table, I witnessed a first-hand account of the body's palpable response to the hands-on application of pressure when targeting the sensitive nerve endings on the feet.

From back problems to digestive upset to hormone imbalances, all symptoms were touched by the power of the foot reflexes. Pain that

I wasn't able to influence through manual therapy was melted away when I addressed the feet. As a mysterious bonus, clients were reporting emotional relief, habit cessation and profound inspiration during our sessions. The work that I had thought was irrelevant was in fact the first real glimpse of what I was looking for all along – a modality that allowed me to bring balance to the entire person. From those first moments, I began to develop my Reflexology practice with the feet as my sole focus (*that was a pun*).

Diving head first into a formal certification in Reflexology and sitting for two national Reflexology exams through the American Reflexology Certification Board, I began to max out my credentials. Still thirsty for more knowledge, I started to explore how others practiced the art and science of foot work. By chance, I came across a small book on foot reading. The book was less than stellar and the content, I would later find, was largely a reprint from the works of others; but a basic idea was conveyed: The reflexes for the physical body aren't the only thing that can be mapped onto the feet. Additional research revealed to me that there was an entire sub-culture of foot assessment that no other Reflexology literature had mentioned.

The painful fact emerged that Reflexology is a myopic technique; only concerned with the hands-on manipulation of the reflexes. The primal idea of press-reflex-fix-issue pervades Reflexology literature and there is little to no mention of assessing those same reflexes – let alone considering the mental/emotional aspect of the feet. Instead, there are only rumored tales of expert Reflexologists who are able to truly see into the body through the foot reflexes after many years of practice – rarely do these Reflexologists explain their approach or document their work. What Reflexology has developed into is a limited definition that defaults to a manual therapy. In some states, Reflexology cannot be practiced without extensive licensure, which further ignores the practical application of assessing the very reflexes they are then licensed to apply pressure to.

I wish to correct this trajectory. Instead of blind technique and operating by routines based on concepts such as press-point-fix-issue, Reflexologists and indeed the general public should be taught foot reading; adding how to appropriately assess the physical and internal signs of stress through the window of the extremities to the conversation. This new approach will emphasize and implement an active dialogue between someone assessing another or self-assessing, facilitated by the theories outlined in this text. Courageously listening to the body's voice is a missing element within the current Reflexology atmosphere. We could dramatically increase the value of Reflexology applications with the addition of assessment, or even creating a consultative approach that does not include manual therapies and relies strictly on lifestyle correction to achieve results is the needed alignment moving forward. Hence, this book was created in an effort to start a new dialogue within the Reflexology community.

The Origins of Reflexology

Essentially, the origins of Reflexology begin with a seminal concept that the body and its parts can be mapped onto the extremities. Different cultures have adopted and transformed this idea to include or exclude the surfaces of the tongue, face, eye, hands, the thumb alone, the feet and other surfaces. Each emergence of the Reflexology theory has its own reasoning and vocabulary behind the mapping diagrams and technique. However, the core idea remains the same: We have access to the whole through the part. A perfect book for this is *Reflexology: Art, Science & History* by Christine Issel, which I will let illuminate the exact dates and timelines independent of this work. We are more focused on the immediate theory of assessment here.

I will not attempt to explain the Eastern variations of Reflexology practice as they are not my purview. However, in the West, the popular re-emergence of Reflexology is credited to Dr. William Fitzgerald who practiced a technique he called *Zone Therapy*. Fitzgerald passed on his work to Dr. Joe Shelby Riley, who then passed it on to Eunice Ingham. Ingham created the modern interpretation of the reflexes on the feet and hands that we know as Reflexology today. Again, here we see the work has evolved to echo the body's likeness on the feet and hands. It is from the work of Ingham's lineage that I initially learned to practice the hands-on technique Reflexology.

The shocker came when foot reading was introduced to the equation as most Reflexology maps only focus on physical reflexes of organs, glands and joints of the body. The integration of foot reading brought forward the missing mental/emotional interpretation of the foot's sections into my practice. I had been trained to focus on reflex locations such as the hip reflexes, the eye and ear reflexes, the lower digestive reflexes, glandular reflexes, etc. Foot reading is the opposite and maps the manifestations of internal stressors such as one's sense of security, family and relationships, career, emotions and mental state.

The two schools of thought are opposite in content, yet both propose a similar teaching. Each of the two schools of Reflexology theory details half of the full picture. One limits itself to mapping the physical body structures, while the other limits itself to the subtle personality traits of a person and coaching someone based on the messages held within the feet. In this tome we will be weaving both perspectives together. Helping you learn to offer both meanings and understand the true interconnected nature of the body. The discussion of the subtle and gross aspects of assessment work together and give a complete story of what is happening on all levels of an individual. Moving into a more holistic framework of how symptoms originate and fine tuning all aspects of the self brings Reflexology into a whole new realm as a craft. Understanding that united perspective, is the message I impart most onto my students.

How we Map the Feet Physically

In anatomical studies, imaginary lines are drawn onto the body to distinguish between major sections based on location, function and structure. Likewise, we divide the feet into major sections through the use of lines we call Guidelines. There are four Guidelines in total, each named after the area where it rests. With these Guidelines we can establish a general overview of how the feet are mapped and where specific physical reflexes are located. Based on this foundation, we will continue to build both physical and mental/emotional meaning onto the outlined sections of the feet.

What will commonly differ from Reflexology school to Reflexology school is reflex location. However, this should not happen. If the foot mirrors the body, then why isn't there one map? The first explanation is that each school's theory is different. Some Reflexology institutions have maps that don't necessarily follow a mirrored body model and the reflex locations are shifted based on lineage (*i.e. this is how we've always done it*). Others slightly deviate their mapping based on copyright laws, which require that no one can copy another person's design even if they are referencing the same theory (*i.e. covering their butt*). The combination of these two deviations creates a lack of standardization, but ideally there should be as close a match between the arrangement of physical anatomy and the arrangement of the foot reflexes as possible.

In the image below, you see the five Horizontal Zones of the foot in all their glory as made clear by the location of the four Guidelines. This will serve as a visual aide as we begin to delve into the location of each reflex zone and outline what body reflexes are located within each section of the foot. However, there is also a strong mental/emotional component to each zone. Beside the physical label of 'Head & Neck' you will see the mental/emotional label of 'Thoughts & Opinions' and so on, in order to display the full interconnection of the internal and external scope of Foot Reading. After detailing the physical location of the reflexes there will be a further description of those subtler interpretations of the zones.

Also in the image below, you see what are known as Vertical Zones. After learning the physical and mental/emotional meaning behind each area of the foot, we then add context through adding these vertical sections to our map. The full name of these sections are Vertical Zones of Influence and they tell us which physical and mental/emotional stressors are influencing a marker to manifest in the feet. All of this information is placed within the picture below to give you a visual aid when learning about the various placement and meanings of the zones. I will continue to clarify these aspects as we go along, but it would behoove you to stare intently at the image below and memorize the following Horizontal and Vertical Zone locations and meanings. It should also be mentioned that the image displays Horizontal Zones on the right foot and Vertical Zones of Influence on the left foot, but both zones are present on each foot. Can you imagine how chaotic the image would be if I combined the two into one graphic? Instead, I separated and color coded them for simplicity. Just make sure you don't let the instructional picture limit you to one side of the story per foot!

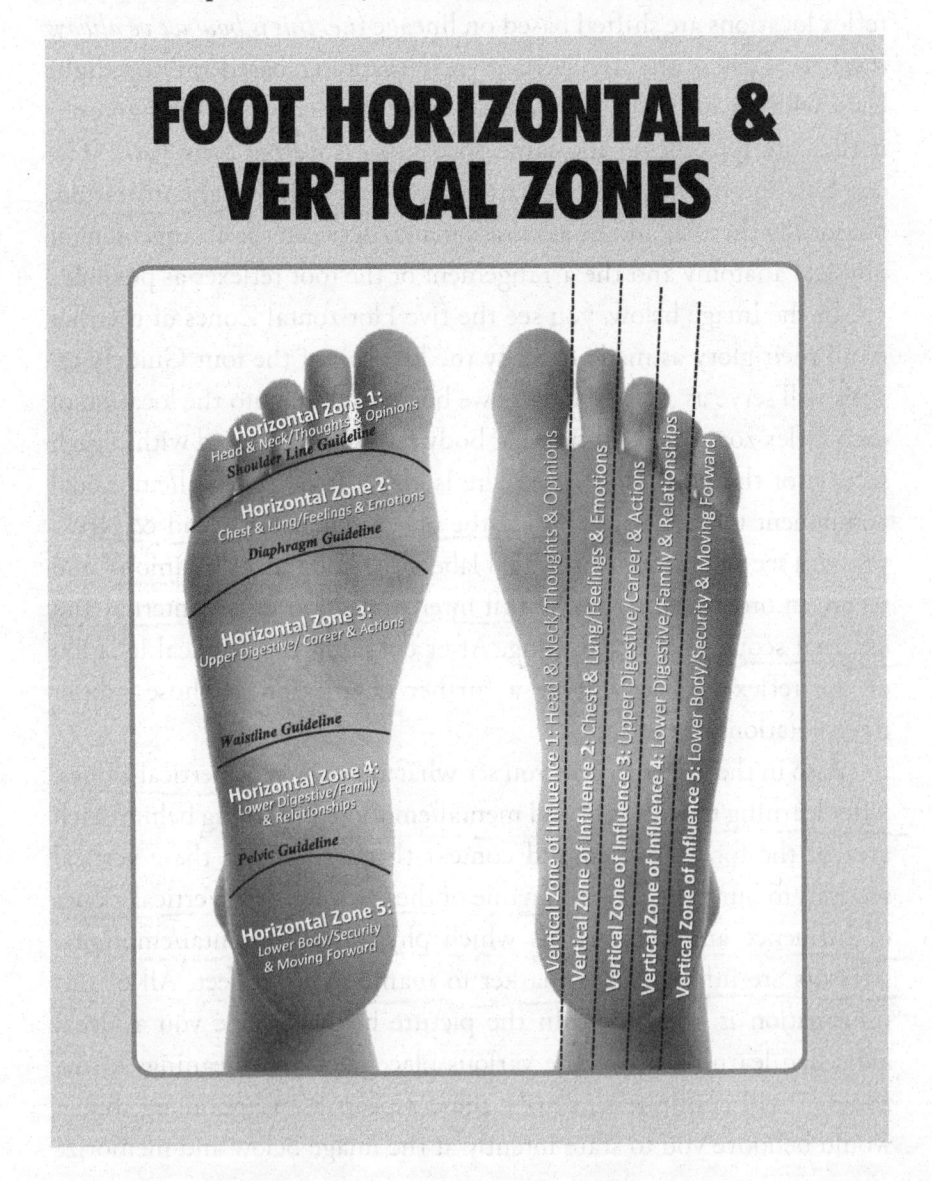

FOOT HORIZONTAL & VERTICAL ZONES

Horizontal Zone 1: Head & Neck/Thoughts & Opinions
Shoulder Line Guideline

Horizontal Zone 2: Chest & Lung/Feelings & Emotions
Diaphragm Guideline

Horizontal Zone 3: Upper Digestive/Career & Actions
Waistline Guideline

Horizontal Zone 4: Lower Digestive/Family & Relationships
Pelvic Guideline

Horizontal Zone 5: Lower Body/Security & Moving Forward

Vertical Zone of Influence 1: Head & Neck/Thoughts & Opinions
Vertical Zone of Influence 2: Chest & Lung/Feelings & Emotions
Vertical Zone of Influence 3: Upper Digestive/Career & Actions
Vertical Zone of Influence 4: Lower Digestive/Family & Relationships
Vertical Zone of Influence 5: Lower Body/Security & Moving Forward

Shoulderline Guideline:

An imaginary line that divides the head and neck structures from the chest, lung and shoulder area. Likewise, dividing the toes from the ball of the foot by drawing a line at the intersection between where the toes grow out from the foot.

Diaphragm Guideline:

An imaginary line that divides the chest, lung and shoulder area from the structures of the upper digestive system and upper core. Likewise, dividing the ball of the foot from the distal (*farther from the body*) arch of the foot by drawing a line where the planted ball of the foot begins to lift into said arch.

Waistline Guideline:

An imaginary line that divides the upper core from the structures of the lower core and pelvic area. Likewise, dividing the proximal (*closer to the body*) arch of the foot from the distal arch of the foot by drawing a line from the proximal head of the 5th metatarsal across the midsection of the arch.

Pelvic Guideline:

An imaginary line that divides the lower core and pelvic structures from the lower body. Likewise, dividing the proximal arch of the foot from the heel by drawing a line where the thick padding of the heel begins to form and plant down from said arch.

These four lines give us a reference point to then map the specific reflex points onto the structures of the foot as they would appear in the body. As you can see by the image above, these Guidelines create sections within the body and the foot. These sections are termed Horizontal Zones and these zones give us an overview of what reflex/body section we are referencing. Especially when reading the feet, speaking in zones gives us shorthand when referring to areas of meaning, such as: "There is a patch of dryness in Horizontal Zone Two, indicating weakness and exhaustion in the chest/lung reflex area."

These zones then give us a baseline vocabulary to communicate our findings with ourselves, people we are reading, and other readers. That being said, the first step of mastering foot reading is to learn the landscape by memorizing these zones and their meanings. We will now expand on the zones by adding the locations of the physical reflexes, but know that we will also associate each zone with a mental/emotional component as well. Without first memorizing the zones we have no context for pinpointing deviations in the reflex tissues. All of the future work in this book is based on learning the zones and what reflexes are contained within.

You will note an asterisk by some of the following reflexes mentioned below. This is due to the mapping variations mentioned earlier. Certain maps may differ in their placement of the following reflex areas, but for our purposes we are using a more exact mapping protocol that mirrors the body. Another important point is that we are dividing the body in half with the right foot representing the right side of the body and the left foot representing the left side of the body. This distinction becomes very important as we map the organs that only appear on one side of the body.

Horizontal Zone One

Location: The Toes
Guideline: Shoulderline
Physical Reflexes Present: All structures of the head, neck and face. Including: Brain, Skull, Sinus, Eyes*, Teeth, Jaw, Ears*, Thyroid, Cervical Spine, Muscles/Bones of the Head and Face

To Reinforce: The toes represent the head and neck. Specifically, the necks of the toes (proximal and middle toe bones, also known as phalanges) represent the neck of the body. The pads of the toes represent the head itself. While each of the toes do represent the head and neck, later in this section we will discuss the meaning behind each individual toe as being influenced by another physical/mental/emotional aspect adding deeper levels to the reading.

Horizontal Zone Two

Location: The Ball of the Foot
Guideline: Shoulderline & Diaphragm
Physical Reflexes Present: Shoulder, Lung, Heart (*more left side*), Ribs, Thymus, Breast, Arm*, Diaphragm (*technically on the Diaphragm Guideline*), Lymph Drainage, Upper Half of Thoracic Spine, Muscles/Bones of the Chest

To Reinforce: Let it be known that as we move from the midline of the body (*medial*) to the outside of the body (*lateral*) we follow the body's structure as well. The heart, which is located more on the left, will have its reflex more on the left center of the foot's ball. Muscles and bones like the pecs and ribs that traverse the expanse of the chest also can be found throughout the entire ball of the foot. The shoulders and their supporting musculature can be found laterally towards the outside edges of the chest areas and so can their reflexes be found more laterally in the ball of the foot with the actual shoulder joint in line with the 5th digit in Horizontal Zone Two.

Horizontal Zone Three

Location: Distal Arch
Guideline: Diaphragm & Waistline
Physical Reflexes Present: Liver (*right foot*), Gallbladder (*right foot*), Pancreas (*more left foot*), Stomach (*left foot*), Spleen (*left foot*), Adrenal, Upper Half of Kidneys, Solar Plexus (*technically on Diaphragm Guideline*), Lower Half of Thoracic Spine, Muscles/Bones of the Upper Core

To Reinforce: Here we see the intricacies of mapping at its finest. The liver is on the right side of the body, while the stomach is on the left. The same is true for the liver's assistant the gallbladder, and the major organ of immunity, the spleen. The pancreas technically expands beyond the midline and only the upper half of the kidneys are present as they straddle the upper and lower halves of the core. Variations can be accounted for in the case of organ rearrangement or benign individualized shifting from the norm.

Horizontal Zone Four

Location: Proximal Arch
Guideline: Waistline & Pelvic
Physical Reflexes Present: Large Intestine (*ascending and half of transverse on right foot; descending, sigmoid and half of transverse on left foot*), Small Intestine, Uterus/Prostate (*medial ankle*), Fallopian Tubes/Vas Deferens (*dorsal ankle*), Ovaries/Testes (*lateral ankle*), Ureters, Bladder, Lower Half of Kidneys, Inguinal Lymph Drainage, Hip Joint (*lateral ankle*), Lumbar Spine, Muscles/Bones of the Lower Core.

To Reinforce: Horizontal Zone Four has the widest variety of reflexes ranging from key joints of mobility to urinary and reproductive organs. All of these placements requires an in depth knowledge of anatomical arrangement. There are reflexes that are more central and those reflexes more outskirt; each corresponding to where it is located within the body. You will also note that the same reflex location is given for the male and female reproductive reflexes. However, they naturally alternate based on the hormonal proclivity of the individual.

Now would be a good time to address removal or transition of the organs and the effect on their reflexes. The physical location stays intact, but the area is altered by how the change is received by the body. Inflammation, scar tissue or emptiness may be present. By far, the most interesting of these changes in the reflexes is organ/gland adaptation. Instead of simply 'going without', the body will often recruit other structures to adapt and pick up the slack for the body to remain in a balanced state to the best of its abilities. Keep your eyes open for clues as to how the body has fully received the alteration.

FOOT READING

Horizontal Zone Five

<u>Location:</u> Heel
<u>Guideline:</u> Pelvic
<u>Physical Reflexes Present:</u> Sciatic Nerve, Sacral Spine, Coccyx, Muscles/Bones of the Legs/Low Body

To Reinforce: Probably the easiest zone to understand, the heel is associated to the lower body in its entirety. So goes the heel, so goes the lower body.

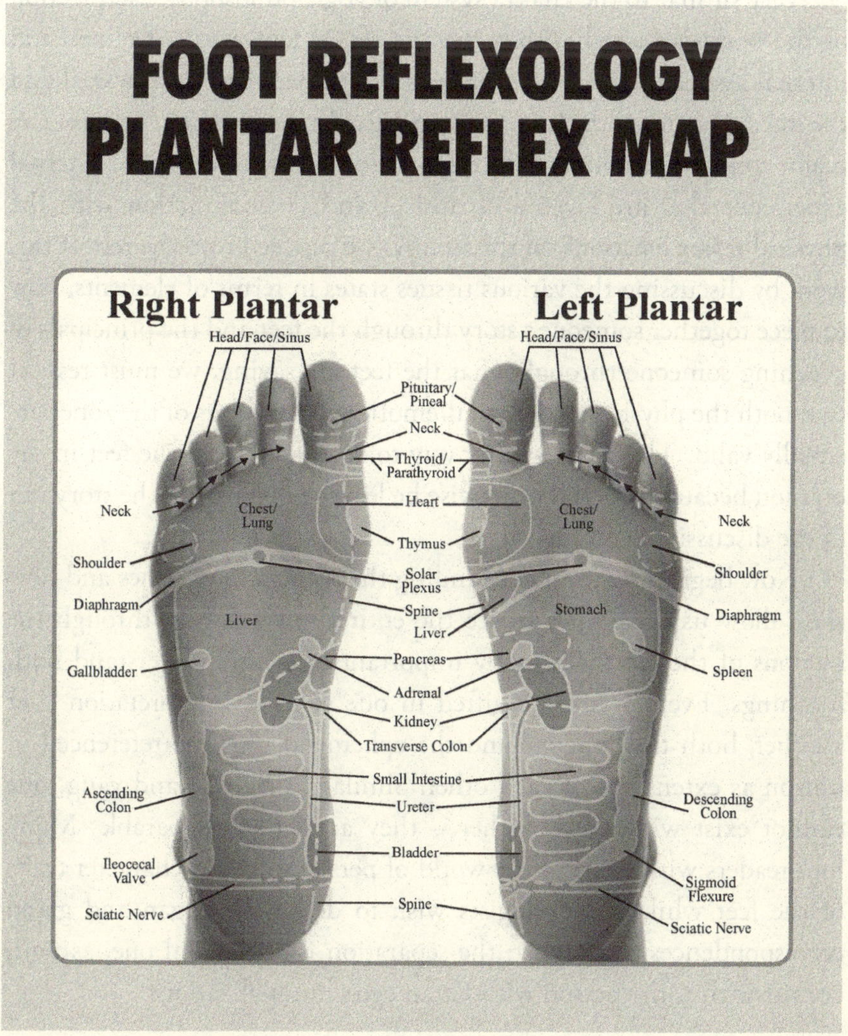

FOOT REFLEXOLOGY PLANTAR REFLEX MAP

Right Plantar
- Head/Face/Sinus
- Neck
- Shoulder
- Diaphragm
- Liver
- Gallbladder
- Ascending Colon
- Ileocecal Valve
- Sciatic Nerve
- Chest/Lung

Left Plantar
- Head/Face/Sinus
- Pituitary/Pineal
- Neck
- Thyroid/Parathyroid
- Heart
- Thymus
- Solar Plexus
- Spine
- Liver
- Pancreas
- Adrenal
- Kidney
- Transverse Colon
- Small Intestine
- Ureter
- Bladder
- Spine
- Chest/Lung
- Stomach
- Neck
- Shoulder
- Diaphragm
- Spleen
- Descending Colon
- Sigmoid Flexure
- Sciatic Nerve

The Mental/Emotional Meaning of the Zones

The biggest impact my work has had on me is the real-time physical validation of internal stress through the feet. Nothing expresses the deepest joy I experience when the feet speak to me in such a real way as to detail the exact mental and emotional state of an individual through seemingly random changes in the tissues of the extremities. There is really nothing like it. This wisdom, I would now like to share with you as the next layer of understanding the zones of the feet.

Very similar to the chakra system of yogic philosophy, each section of the body is paired with a specific set of key words, feelings and internal associations which serve as a bridge between the physical and the internal states of the human experience. In foot reading, we have five major zones or centers that correspond to five major realms of internal experience that are layered on top of and in conjunction with the physical reflex locations on the feet. As we proceed into the rest of this work by discussing the various tissues states in terms of elements, how to piece together someone's story through the feet and the principals of coaching someone through what the feet are saying, we must respect that both the physical and mental/emotional meanings of the zones are equally valid. There is no other way to accurately read the feet in my opinion because you will otherwise be leaving one half of the story out of the discussion.

Now beginning to understanding the principals of zones and how they allow us the ability to see the entirety of a person through the sections of the feet, it is vastly important to clearly understand both meanings. Even if you are gifted in one style of interpretation over another, both the concrete and the ephemeral must be referenced in unison as extensions of each other. Similar to the yin and yang, one cannot exist without the other – they are truly inseparable. Many foot readers wish to be in the world of personality and character traits of the feet while Reflexologists wish to detail the organ and gland correspondences of the feet; the separation is a fictional one, as both coexist within the person without an ego's rationalizations.

FOOT READING

Horizontal Zone One

Location: The Toes
Guideline: Shoulderline
Mental/Emotional Meaning: Thoughts and Opinions

To Reinforce: Yes, the toes represent the head and neck, but the head and neck is the center of our mental state and how we vocalize our mind-musings. When considering the meaning of distorted toes, stubbed digits and nails that become unruly, the place to look is within the energetic significance of what is floating between the ears of the person in question. Not just the nature of one's thoughts, but how those thoughts are then expressed or not expressed appropriately. A clear and well-oiled mind is a force of great significance – the absence of those qualities has a very real effect on the body's state.

Just like with the physical reflex locations in the toes, there is a difference between the neck reflexes being in the necks of the toes and the actual head reflexes being in the pads of the toes. With the subtle interpretation of toe meaning, the necks of the toes relay how one expresses one's thoughts while the pads and nails of the toes represent the overall quality of those opinions.

Horizontal Zone Two

Location: The Ball of the Foot
Guideline: Shoulderline & Diaphragm
Mental/Emotional Meaning: Feelings and Emotions

To Reinforce: Both primal and complex, how we feel on a moment to moment basis drastically swings the pendulum of wellness from one extreme to another; knowing that both the physical and internal heart rest within the ball of the feet is the significance of this center. The individual fluctuations and their meaning will vary based on the tissues states we witness in this area that will be discussed deeper into the book.

Not all emotions are watery or fiery. Instead, each feeling has its own corresponding visual and textural set of identifiers.

Horizontal Zone Three

Location: Distal Arch
Guideline: Diaphragm & Waistline
Mental/Emotional Meaning: Career and Actions

To Reinforce: The combustive and emulsifying alchemy of the upper digestive system is home to our internal purpose and drive to succeed in the world via the vehicle of our contributions. The job we do is the most relevant part of that momentum, but all possible daily actions we take including schooling, volunteer work and vocational living are also grouped into this category. Horizontal Zone Three represents our driving force, or lack thereof, that propels us to act and make a difference while enduring the purifying heat of our activities. Knots in the stomach and congestion in the liver are directly related to our sense of this career and actions dynamic, so too does this center of the foot distort under stress related to one's work.

Horizontal Zone Four

Location: Proximal Arch
Guideline: Waistline & Pelvic
Mental/Emotional Meaning: Family and Relationships

To Reinforce: Our family unit is often the most tender and conditional space we hold within our lattice of self. Whether our inner circle is connected by blood or choice, both are organic. The reference here is to whom we give our attention to. The support, exchange and arrangement of those relationships create the shape and condition of Horizontal Zone Four. When we examine the physical bones of this zone we find that they make up the most lifted part of our arch, the part of us that literally puts the spring in our step – as natural association, the same function is sought of our immediate circle of friends and family.

Horizontal Zone Five

<u>Location:</u> Heel
<u>Guideline:</u> Pelvic
<u>Mental/Emotional Meaning:</u> Sense of Security and Moving Forward

To Reinforce: Physically, Horizontal Zone Five has the simplest meaning; with no complex array of organs. Internally, there is a complexity of having a balanced foundation that is present. How we are moving forward, or not moving forward, forges the quality of our sense of stability. Do I feel safe? Do I know what is coming next or how to make my next move? These questions at the base of our hierarchy of needs also affect the base of our bodies.

Moving from our Guidelines, to our physical reflexes, to our mental/emotional meanings creates an excellent starting point for the beginning foot reader to experiment. Comparing your previous life experiences is also helpful to create a frame of reference based on your own timelines and symptoms. As we progress in our studies, the concepts in this chapter will be referred to constantly. Memorizing the basics at this juncture is essential. However, allow your exploration to resemble a game. Have fun with this new knowledge that even the most seemingly insignificant foot issue has meaning. Raw facts are important, but curiosity is what will ingrain into your memory the live instances of foot reading you come across.

Vertical Zones of Influence

In assessment there is great significance to the exact location of symptoms in a particular Horizontal Zone. This significance is mapped on the feet by creating five Vertical Zones with one Vertical Zone in line with each toe. We then distribute the same physical and internal meanings of the Horizontal Zones along the Vertical Zones to create a complete grid system on which all symptoms will be read. Although it seems complicated at first, with repetition there is an easy correlation and logical order to the Vertical Zones of Influence.

Vertical Zones were the major mapping system used by Dr. William Fitzgerald in his technique of Zone Therapy, although no in depth meaning was given. Fitzgerald viewed these vertical columns to be lines of influence and any organ, gland or structure to be in their path would feel the holistic effect of stimulus to any other place along the same zone. Today, I define the Vertical Zones as influencing which means that they tell us, based on where the symptom is located, what body systems and internal stressors helped to manifest that particular distortion in the foot's tissues. Where Horizontal Zones provide the map of the physical and internal states on the feet, the Vertical Zones give us a deeper context for the significance of a symptoms location.

In this way, a foot reader may understand a symptoms appearance within a representative reflex zone and read its physical/internal meaning, but the reader can also know what physical/internal factors created the symptom by gridding the location using Vertical Zones. I have found this particular use of Vertical Zones to be scarily accurate and encourage you to play with the following mapping technology with the intention of adding an even more profound layer to this work of reading the feet.

Vertical Zone One

Location: In Line with the Big Toe
Physical Influences: All reflexes found in Horizontal Zone One
Mental/Emotional Influence: Thoughts and Opinions

To Reinforce: A symptom falling in line with the big toe falls into Vertical Zone One. This means there is a direct influence of the physical reflexes located in the head and neck space, but also a heavy theme of mental stress added to the meaning. This also means that the big toe itself, being in Horizontal One and Vertical Zone One, is truly the lighthouse to for all things related to the head and neck.

FOOT READING

Vertical Zone Two

<u>Location:</u> In Line with the Second Toe
<u>Physical Influences:</u> All reflexes found in Horizontal Zone Two
<u>Mental/Emotional Influence:</u> Feelings and Emotions

To Reinforce: As you well know, feelings are powerful. In this case, the physical and internal aspects of the chest are involved when we find markers in line with the second toe. Especially when we see heightened activity in the ball of the foot (Horizontal Zone Two) in line with the second toe (Vertical Zone Two), there is always a serious emotional flavor to all symptomology present within the feet.

Vertical Zone Three

<u>Location:</u> In Line with the Third Toe
<u>Physical Influences:</u> All reflexes found in Horizontal Zone Three
<u>Mental/Emotional Influence:</u> Career and Actions

To Reinforce: Many people don't see this influence coming, but I see it in my practice almost every day. The upper GI tract is a very powerful influencer and so is our work environment. Should you see dysfunction in the center zone of the foot, you know that both the upper core and one's career are at play.

Vertical Zone Four

<u>Location:</u> In Line with the Fourth Toe
<u>Physical Influences:</u> All reflexes found in Horizontal Zone Four
<u>Mental/Emotional Influence:</u> Family and Relationships

To Reinforce: Sensitivity is the name of this Vertical Zone's game. There is no touchier subject than one's home life and the individuals that may or may not be pulling their weight. Tread compassionately, yet firmly with this Vertical Zone and symptoms in line with the fourth toe.

Vertical Zone Five

Location: In Line with the Fifth Toe
Physical Influences: All reflexes found in Horizontal Zone Five
Mental/Emotional Influence: Sense of Security and Moving Forward

To Reinforce: All symptoms in line with the little toe have the essence of the need to move forward and are directly related to the lower body reflexes. This zone does have a flare for dramatic symptoms so be warned, you won't be able to misinterpret this zone.

Test your Knowledge

Combining the above Vertical Zones with the already discussed Horizontal Zones is quite simple. All you need to do is state the meanings of the Horizontal Zone and say that it is being *influenced by* the meanings of the Vertical Zone. This creates a concrete statement of interpretation that can be refined and expounded upon based on factors like other symptoms present, timelines and adjectives; all of which we will be discussing later in this book. For now, begin to create mock scenarios in your mind to help you rehearse the meanings of the Horizontal and Vertical Zones such as the ones below:

- *What is the physical meaning of a symptom at Horizontal Zone One & Vertical Zone Four?*
- *What is the mental/emotional meaning of a symptom at Horizontal Zone Three & Vertical Zone Two?*
- *What is the physical meaning of a symptom at Horizontal Zone Two & Vertical Zone Five?*
- *What is the mental/emotional meaning of a symptom at Horizontal Zone Five & Vertical Zone Three?*
- *What is the physical meaning of a symptom at Horizontal Zone Two & Vertical Zone One?*
- *What is the mental/emotional meaning of a symptom at Horizontal Zone Four & Vertical Zone Three?*

FOOT READING

Additional Nuances when Mapping the Feet

Top of the Foot vs. Bottom of the Foot

To be clear, the physical reflexes are what I like to call *through and through*. This means the same reflexes that are located on the top of the foot can be found on the bottom of the foot. Now, there are some hairs to split here. If we are thinking of the foot as a representation of the body, our body has a front and a back. Therefore, the foot's top or dorsal surface would be the back of the body and the sole or plantar surface would be the front of the body. A good analogy would be in Horizontal Zone Two; the ball of the foot would represent the chest, breast, pec and structures in the front of that body zone while the top of the foot would be more the upper back muscles and shoulder blade reflexes.

There are also additional meanings to consider from a mental/emotional perspective. When you can look down onto feet that are resting comfortably on the floor, you can only see the tops. This dorsal surface represents traits that the outside world can see clearly and that are not hidden. Contra, when the feet are at rest you cannot see the soles of the feet and the plantar surface of each foot represents more internal or hidden traits that the outside world does not normally see. I will notice a dramatic difference in some feet when looking on top vs. bottom, while others seem consistent on both sides – just an added level to your assessments.

Recently, I had a colleague of mine explain that they were having a terrible skin irritation between their second and third toes. After confirming that he was indeed experiencing sinus irritation due to acid reflex symptoms over the last week and that he was indeed fired up about moving from his current job that he hated to a new opportunity, we then peered deeper into the feet. Looking at the foot, I could not tell from the outside that there was such an irritation. It wasn't until they manually separated that I was able to see the red and irritated tissues. This would mean that my colleague was able to hide his irritation from the world, but it was still very present internally.

Left Foot vs. Right Foot

As you've already learned, the feet contain a map of the body that is exact, but we have a right foot and a left foot. Each foot contains half of the body with the right foot containing the right side of the body's reflexes and the left foot containing the left side of the body's reflexes. That differentiation becomes very important as you begin to uncover symptomology in the reflexes. If a client reports pain on the right side of the low back, but the low back reflexes on the left side are swollen then we know the source of the pain is more on the left side of the body.

Now we add the internal difference between markers appearing on the left foot versus the right foot. When assessing the mental/emotional meanings of the reflexes, all markers on the right foot are associated with the past and all markers on the left foot are associated with the present. I tried to personally dispute this fact in the beginning as it seemed too subtle of a distinction to make. However, I have found the right and left feet being associated with the past and present respectively to be very true.

This brings up a key difference between more esoteric and intuitive reading of the extremities, such as the hands, and the art and science of foot reading. We do not look into the future. Instead, we are only concerned with the present state of an individual on a physical and mental/emotional level. In regards to the past, we see lingering physical and internal stress that is stuck in the person's current state. I will frequently tell my students: If it is not in the feet, it doesn't exist. This is true for present and past complaints. However, if there is a marker on the right foot you need to recognize that the past issue associated with that marker has not been released.

Gait and Walking Patterns

One of my favorite class activities during our Reflexology certification that I teach at the institute is our field trip to the mall. During this group exercise, we all sit at a table in the food court and watch people walk. The observations we all have really put foot reading into perspective and I encourage you to try this in any heavily foot-traffic area. Why not bring a few friends and make it a walk watching party?!

The goal of this is to see the varying ways people throw their weight onto the feet when they walk. From a physical perspective, we can see someone putting massive pressure on specific physical reflexes that can be easily interpreted as putting excess pressure on the associated joints or organs. When we observe the same walk from a subtle aspect, there is a display of where someone is placing the most energy in their life based on which zone and which foot is bearing the most weight while walking.

Another pearl of wisdom I give to my students is that your job as an extremity assessment expert is to know more about the client's story than they do. From the moment they walk through the door, your eyes should be combing over the finer details of any visible markers and their gait, listening to the words they are using and piecing together the body's message. Non-verbal cues are what foot readers thrive on and how someone walks into their session can be the first clue you pick up on.

Zooming In

Occasionally, I will see a marker that appears very significant and seems to be drawing a majority of my attention on a particular extremity. In addition to being visually striking, I will notice that the marker seems to be hovering on the tissues in a way that makes me think there is more to the story. This is when I will impose a zoomed in version of the Horizontal and Vertical Zone map into the Horizontal Zone where the marker is located. It's an advanced technique that definitely requires a mastery of the zones and mapping principles, but a powerful addition to your Foot Reading toolkit.

As an example, I'll see an injury in Horizontal Zone Two that is situated mid-way down a Vertical Zone that seems to be (*in the case of a zoomed in map*) also in Horizontal Zone Three. Seeing the marker with this additional meaning would prompt me to add the physical and mental/emotional meaning of the upper digestive reflexes on that side and the past/present state of that person's career stress. Of course this is very nuanced work and technically advanced, but some markers will just seem to be saying more than the broad definitions associated with a zoomed out map.

A perfect example of this technique is on the nails of the toes, which are microcosms in and of themselves. Nail issues, injuries and deformities' are common and all have the standard Horizontal Zone One interpretation, but when you zoom in to the individual nail there is a world inside that surface like no other. Each nail will sometimes tell a story based on the ridges, dips and dynamic formations present. A whole session could be done on interpreting a single nail! Zooming in on individual markers can deepen your work to an unfathomable level; provided you know the map inside and out.

Section Recap

- Foot assessment is a **cross-cultural practice** found throughout the world.
- The recent emergence of Reflexology theory in the West includes figureheads such as **Dr. William Fitzgerald, Joe Shelby Riley and Eunice Ingham.**
- Foot Reading is a practice that integrates the location of **both physical and mental/emotional** reflex areas.
- The four Guidelines that help us map the feet are: **Shoulderline, Diaphragm, Waistline and Pelvic.**
- There are **Five Horizontal Zones** which help us locate physical and mental/emotional areas of stress on the feet as they appear in the body.
- There are **Five Vertical Zones of Influence** which help us understand factors that influence various stressors to manifest.
- Additional nuances to consider when reading the feet are: **Top vs. Bottom, Left vs. Right, Walking Patterns and Zooming In.**

Elements of a Symptom

Venturing deeper into the jungles of foot reading requires a firmer understanding of assessment vocabulary. We have created a map of the landscape by using the zones and their meanings, but we need to add the words that describe in detail what the types of terrain we might find during a session. If we were to give an account of our findings to another, we need to use a series of commonly understood terms that resonate easily and convey the basic concept of what we have seen. For this purpose, we will use the four major Western elements: Earth, Air, Fire and Water.

Elements are used similarly in other assessment systems. Ayurveda and Traditional Chinese Medicine (TCM) are two popular examples, although different in their theories. Taking a hint from each of their systems, I began to associate the four elements of Earth, Air, Fire and Water with the symptoms I found when reading feet. I also started slipping in elemental language when conveying my findings to my clients. This was a tremendous success and I have compiled my thoughts on this method in this chapter. The goal of this material is learning how to describe what you find during a foot reading assessment in a clear and simple language that can be universally understood while staying accurate to the physical and mental/emotional symptom being described.

We will be discussing each element in relation to constitution and associated symptoms. Constitution refers to one's default physical and mental/emotional makeup. Associated symptoms would be conditions such as dryness, callousing, pain and swelling. My approach uses an element's qualities in relation to a person's personality, physical makeup and the nature of various symptoms you will find during an assessment. We call these visual and textural signs 'markers', which relates to a strong elemental presence across the foot tissues. Describing the marker in elemental terms is an easy way to relay the body's message to the client, but also allows you to better understand the relationship between the various systems and symptoms of the body.

For example, the center of heat in the body is Horizontal Zone Three – the center of combustive digestion and metabolism. There is a certain level of heat and tension you would expect to find here as the body chemically and manually breaks down and filters nutrients. If you see puffiness and paleness in the tissues of this zone, then feedback can be given as to this center holding onto excess Water (*puffiness and paleness*). This is how we would use elemental language to convey and assess the markers in the feet. In the next chapter we will put all of the mapping and symptomology together within a solid statement, but for now we are continuing to build the language we will use.

Earth
Density, Width and Growth

The character of Earth as an element in nature brings to mind nutrient rich soils, staggering mountains and magnificently ordered structures like crystals that seem to be frozen in time. To better understand this element, we can look to some of its natural traits that allow us to define how we would see someone with heavy Earth qualities within their physical and internal makeup. As a rule, the major physical association with the element of Earth is **Width**. This refers to the wideness or breadth of the foot's structures and of the foot itself. Width is the sign of having vast amounts of physical resources, like rich soil, at the person's disposal. Width can then be thought of as being a physical trait that marks endurance and perseverance.

Along with width, there is a high level of density in the bones of the foot. You will notice that the bones themselves are rigid and have grown together like a grove of trees, none able to budge as their roots and branches (*ligaments*) have also become hard and intertwined. This combination of density, stiffness and width gives us the image of a mountainous foot that is indeed strong and stable. Almost taking on a square or blockish shape, earthen feet are easy to spot because of their predicable corners highlighted by the shape of their prominent bones.

The individual with an Earth constitution will have both physical and internal qualities known to natural Earth: steadfastness, heaviness and a supportive disposition. Steadfastness can be positively viewed as dependability, reliability and consistency, but can easily unbalance into traits of stubbornness, rigidity and getting stuck in a rut. Heaviness is an overarching quality of both the person and the tissues of the Earth constitution with phrases like 'heavy set' and 'big boned' being used to describe their constitution; note that I am not referring to actual fat content or being plump in shape (*which would be associated with the Water element*), but a true denseness within the stature itself. Support is the trait valued by those who have an earthy person in their life. Earth has both the stamina to get the job done over the long haul and the true desire to help where they can.

Common Earth Symptomology by Zone

Horizontal Zone One

Sizeable Toes – Increased width relays a larger amount of resources, both physically and internally. When all the toes, or specific toes (*refer to Vertical Zone meaning*), have a wider shape there is clear Earth influences at play. The wider size means more energy is available in the reflexes of the head and neck as well as one's thoughts and opinions.

Hairy Toes – Body hair is a protective mechanism in all respects, regardless where it is placed. Hair falls under the growth category of the Earth element and is the dense protective covering of the zones where it is present. The caveat to this marker is the question: Why does this area need protecting? The answer can be found in interpreting what other constitutional elements and markers are present, but the body produces hair when it feels the need to guard that reflex area. Which toes have hair is significant, especially when considering Vertical Zones as not all toes will have hair on them. This marker is more mental/emotional than physical as the toe hair is protecting the person's ability to vocalize that Vertical Zone's qualities; such as thoughts about career (3rd *toe*) or thoughts about moving forward (5th *toe*).

Hardening/Callousing of Toenails – Many people believe that a hardening or callousing of the toe nails is a sign of fungus. I disagree as true nail fungus is normally black and necrotic in color. When the nails become large (*growth*) and calloused (*density*) there is a very different meaning. Hardening and vertical growth of the nail is a hardening and protective layering of the physical soft tissues within the head and face – specifically the eyes, sinuses and gums/teeth. Internally, so go the nails so goes the mind. Symptom-ridden nails that are hardened and layered are a sign of a stagnant and over-crowded mind. Individual nails have meaning to further clarify, but there is a direct correlation between one's mental state and the nails.

Ingrown Toenails – In addition to the above associations with the nails, including eyes, sinus, gums/teeth and one's mental state, when any nail grows inward there is a derailment on all levels of the head space. As summarized by thoughts and physical tissues that are growing out of control and continue to painfully deviate off track.

Hammer Toes – Defined as a toe whose first two phalanges create an upward point, but the tip of the toe still points forward. This is a sign of neck misalignments and of opinions that are being withheld. The nuance of a hammered toe versus a clawed toe, is that there is still a level of openness in this condition and indicates more of a compensation pattern then a full collapse or withdrawal of the Horizontal/Vertical Zone in question.

Claw Toes – When a toe's shape draws in completely and the tip of the toe is pointing into the ground, this is a true claw toe. A structural collapse in the headspace and a kyphotic curling in of the neck and head tissues is the physical meaning of this symptom. Internally, this toe is more difficult to coach out of hiding because defensive tendencies are high. Large amounts of physical and internal stress that is not handled properly will result in the type of retraction found in a fully clawed toe. I have found the second toe to be particularly prone to this condition, which would indicate a collapse of the head, neck and chest dynamic and an internal withdrawal of one's thoughts about how they are feeling.

Leaning/Wrapping Toes – Like the Leaning Tower of Pisa, certain toes can seem to tilt. In extreme cases they can crash into or overtake another toe. This process is fascinating and represents structural deviations in the head, neck, thoughts and opinions. As the lean of a toe gains intensity and begins to shove, wrap and stunt other toes there is a clear invasion happening within the Vertical Zones involved; the greater the lean the stronger the misalignment.

Callousing of the Toes – Everyone's favorite topic, I know, but callousing needs to be understood as the quintessential Earth marker. Hardness, denseness and rigidity at its finest, a callous is strategically placed to indicate where tissues that have become immobile and protective. Commonly, there will be a strong callous at the inner base of the big toe, but not always; this indicates stiffness at the base of the skull. Callouses in the toes indicate a hardening of thought, which toe is significant when you begin to build the story, but the general meaning is a stiff or rigid set of opinions.

Horizontal Zone Two

Wide Ball of the Foot – General wideness in the ball of the foot is common to see – very common in fact. Just as general width indicates large amounts of energy and resources, we then apply the meaning of the ball of the foot to that vastness. Physically, the chest, lung and shoulder reflexes are pronounced, meaning that all of these physical structures will have more weight, but will also be the source of greatest felt tension within the body i.e. chronic complaints of tight upper back and shoulders. Since Horizontal Zone Two dually represents one's feelings and emotions, there is a wide array of feelings within wide-ball individuals that is unique to this marker.

Ball of the Foot Callousing – A popular place for callousing to hang out is within the ball of the foot, sometimes to a painful degree, but pain is a different elemental marker. Here we will see overall stiff and guarded tendencies in the chest, lungs, shoulders, feelings and emotions. A word of warning about general callousing – no amount of shaving a callous will cause it to disappear. Callousing is not brought on by shoes or activity, but by the interconnected intelligence of the nervous system. The best way to soften a callous is to soften the physical and internal aspects where the callous is present. Use your map! This is especially true for the more emotional callousing in Horizontal Zone Two.

Baby Bunion – The lesser known sibling of the classic bunion, but still recognized as a bump that irritates and that people tend to find unsightly. Found in line with the 5th digit (*little toe*) at the lateral edge of Horizontal Zone Two, this bump is situated over the joint of the shoulder reflex giving it a direct physical meaning of shoulder deviations. A prominent, hardened bump indicating that the shoulder itself has become rather large and locked. Emotionally, this bump can be associated with an increased need to shoulder burdens or the struggles of bottled up emotions regarding how to move forward.

The Classic Bunion – Found at the joint between the first metatarsal and the proximal phalanx of the big toe, this studly protrusion of the joint is an adaptation to disperse pressure pushed into the feet from higher up in the body's chain of command. Physically and emotionally, there is a similar meaning along the lines of bottled up pressure. Decompressing a bunion growth can be done, but there is a high level of self-care and self-awareness that is needed. Bunion sufferers have been conditioned over time to suppress their feelings – the larger the bunion, the greater the emotional pressure. Releasing said bunions requires that the individual rewire their ability to discharge excess feelings in a healthy way. Likewise, if this is not done then the bunion will continue to grow and wreak havoc as a marker of the undealt with issues.

Horizontal Zone Three

<u>Rigidity</u> – A quality that I find fascinating about this zone in relation to Earth symptomology is that it is prone to becoming very congested and densified. Physically, this would be a clogging of the upper digestive reflexes with the left side being stomach/spleen/pancreas reflex territory and the right side being liver/gallbladder reflex territory. I will often find one side more densified than the other, so assessing each side thoroughly is needed here. Internally, this marker represents a backlog of issues at work that are not being processed; as if the energy of productivity has been overburdened and halted for some reason. Pay attention to the vertical zones here as well and they will give you the defining clues to interpret the message further.

<u>Dorsal Bone Bump</u> – My absolute favorite marker of all time is the dorsal bumps on the tops of the feet. Why? Because its meaning has become so clear to me over time and many of my clients have found tremendous value in this marker's guidance, I also happen to have this marker pop up on occasion. When you see a pronounced bone growth on the tops of the feet it is a sign of physical malnutrition and anemic tendencies. Basically, the body isn't getting the caloric intake it needs and/or is burning through what nutrition is being given too quickly. When this marker is on one foot, but not another then we take into consideration the physical reflexes present as they are very different and could indicate true anemia or situational anemia.

Internally, this marker is also very interesting. Mirroring a physical sense of hunger, this mental/emotional marker stands for the person having a seemingly bottomless desire to achieve. The drive to make a difference, get ahead and have an impact (*all career/action related*) is strong, but no matter how hard they work nothing seems to satisfy.

The endless pursuit of success is strongly linked with this bone pronouncement. Reminding these individuals that work will always be there tomorrow, that it is not your job to single-handedly save the world and that getting burnt out serves no one, are all important messages to convey in the presence of this marker.

Anemia Bump Story: The first time I nailed the meaning of this marker was with a client who had a very large bump on the top of their right foot. There was no reason for it to be there and my curiosity was peaked. Upon asking about the mystery bump, my client related that it would sometimes get red and painful, but largely went unnoticed. I then relayed the bumps meaning as being situated over the liver reflex and if he had any type of liver condition.

At that point my client's face lit up with surprise and they relayed that they indeed had a diagnosed form of anemia that was largely under control now. Flabbergasted, but still relaying how accurate the assessment was, I then added the internal meaning of past career/work actions being seen as deficient. Amazed again, my client added that their boss was constantly unimpressed with their work and nothing seemed to be good enough despite being the most qualified and innovative person on the development team. This lead my client to feeling like they were constantly playing catchup.

This experience was when I began to solidify the meaning of the bump on the top of the foot. Now, I always share the meaning of this marker with clients who have it as a potential contributing factor to their current state of dis-ease. Having this marker myself, I am always on the lookout for my bumps coming to the surface; for me this is just one way my body tries to get me to slow down and enjoy the life I have created for myself.

Horizontal Zone Four

Collapsed Medial Ankle – As if the structure of the foot has melted, this bone shape has formed from a nervous system that has collapsed in the lower core – the direction of this collapse in a medial orientation is extremely significant. The medial ankle is home to the reflexes for the central pelvis, including the reproductive, bladder, muscular and boney structures of that area; often found in people who have a weakened pelvic floor. There is an internal sense of the family and relationship dynamic surrounding this person also having collapsed and no longer holding them in proper alignment. Both physically and internally, one's core has collapsed with the needed assistance of an internal and external support system.

Callousing – Just the other day I worked on someone who had Horizontal Zone Four completely calloused on the plantar (*bottom*) surface. Their arch was perfectly formed and the excuse was given that they rarely wore shoes, but the rest of the foot was decidedly not calloused. Again, making the case for a unique manifestation that is present to indicate a specific set of symptomology, we can relate the lower digestive reflexes becoming hardened and stagnant; a similar case would be made for the hardening over of their family/relationship dynamic. When this marker is present there are constipation and colon hardening aspects along with a defensive or protective tendency in one's core relationships.

Locked Ankles – So go the ankles so goes the hips. As a general understanding of Horizontal Zone Four there is an immediate correlation with the hips and pelvis. Locking here would indicate locking in the pelvic structures. Stiffness and immobility would also be present within their family/relationship dynamics. It is always best to physically and internally consider which ankle is stiffer. If the right side has solidified but the left has not then there was an infection of Earth energy within the body and relationships, while the opposite with left locked and right freed would mean a current densifying of that same dynamic.

The Arch – Ahh, the arch. A favorite money making topic for Podiatry and shoe companies, but the shape of the arch contains a very different conversation to a Reflexologist who is actively engaged in assessment. The medial arch contains the reflexes for the spine; cervical spine in the big toe, thoracic spine along the first metatarsal bone in medial Horizontal Zone Three and Four, lumbar spine as the lifted arch cushioning the navicular area, with the medial heel representing the sacral spine and coccyx. The height of the arch located in Horizontal Zone Four, like how the largest natural curve is in the lumbar spine. Fallen arches need to be evaluated independently as to where the falling has happened and to what degree. I have met MANY people who assume their arches are flat, high, fallen or perfectly normal when in fact they are not. This crux requires that you visually assess each arch individually and not take someone's word for it, as they have not seen the amount of feet you will have to correctly evaluate. The assessment will not fit them if they are wrong about the state of their own arch.

Arches that have lost their shape in any way relay a structural deviation of the spine column vertebrae. The spinal column represents one's core thoughts and opinions about each Horizontal Zone where it is present or one's 'back bone' of beliefs in that zone's meaning. Structural deviation in the foot's arch is a deviation of the fundamental internal structure that someone has come to rely on about that area of their life. A high arch creates an over-compression, heightened support and an overly curved spine. A low or flattened arch is a spine with no stable (*key word is 'stable'*) curvature and the constant need to be lifted up or supported by others outside of the themselves – high arches are fiercely independent by contrast. Always thinking in terms of how the earthy quality of the arch is behaving to better interpret this area of the foot as a key personality and structural component.

Horizontal Zone Five

<u>Wide Heels</u> – We've discussed width before in terms of having an excess amount of resources and that is true with the heels in Horizontal Zone Five as well. This marker being present will give insight into the lower body of that person being very sturdy and somewhat large. On the other hand, there is an internal aspect of being very grounded and rooted. I often find that this marker bodes well for financial security

specifically, as a side effect of a person constantly broadening their base of support. Measuring this marker in relation to the width of the other zones will also be helpful as the contrast would reveal volumes about strengths and weaknesses. However, if the entire foot has that wide, blockish shape then the heel being wide would fit right in to an overall Earth constitution.

<u>Calloused Heels</u> – No, not everyone has calloused heels. However, the tissues are naturally thick in this zone because the lower body has the most physical thickness. That being said, when callousing erupts onto the heels, there is a present rigidity in the lower body reflexes. Callousing as defensiveness relays an almost fight or flight tendency regarding someone's sense of security; their body has put up a wall to protect an area that feels too sensitive.

The Heel Story: One of my favorite stories to tell about the heels happened to me personally when I was taking the last Reflexology workshop I needed to get the required hours for the American Reflexology Certification Board's national exam. I had been waiting for six months to take that class. Honestly, I was over it. I was so ready to just get it done and to submit my paperwork ASAP. The morning of the first day I was taking my shower and washing my feet when the heel of my left foot began to slough off skin. Never having experienced this before; I was puzzled. Beginning to now scrub vigorously at the molting skin, it just kept coming off and there was no stopping it. There was no pain, no discoloration, no sign that it was there before, just a mass exodus of layer upon layer of heel skin.

Later, learning about the left heel's significance in relation to the present internal stressor of moving forward and taking the next steps, the connection was obvious. My body was releasing the physical and emotional buildup of tissues that I had accumulated from waiting for this class over the past six months. To this day, when I tell this story I get multiple students relaying similar mass shedding experiences that have happened to them around periods of great change.

An Overall Note on Warts, Tags and Moles...

Growths are a very charged topic in medicine. The average person spends good money to have things removed and treated, only for them to come back. The shame and self-consciousness of having bumps that shouldn't be there also fuels the aggressive journey to do away with mystery lumps. From an elemental perspective, these growths fall into the Earth category as they are extracellular growths that are presenting an excess within the tissues. Many variations and names exist for these little buggers, so let's define what I mean by warts and moles to go along with the elemental association of Earth.

When looking from a marker perspective, there are quite a few differences in the common bump that appears on the surface of the skin. To be sure we are looking at a true Earth marker the wart or mole must be a raised growth on top of the skin. This is different from conditions under the skin such as acne, boils and even plantar warts (*which are more of a hole in the skin and are cave-like*). A true wart, tag or mole may appear individually or in a cluster, the trick is to first identify that it is truly an extra growth on top of the skin and not another condition; then we can interpret correctly.

Growths are growths and their behavior over specific reflexes indicates the body's propensity to grow extra cells within that reflex area. Most warts, tags and moles are stationary, unmoving and are relatively boring. These types are simply a warning sign that there is additional cell activity within the area in question. Mentally/Emotionally, where the growth is located also means excess activity in the meaning of that area. When there is a singular growth, there is a singular issue. Clusters represent a cluster of issues within that Horizontal and Vertical Zone's meaning. Additional coaching questions may be asked to further identify the backstory of the growth(s). Color is also significant, but belongs to another element.

Two Wart Stories: I have had many clients come in to see me with specific warts or clusters, but two extreme cases stick out in my mind. The first was a client with a large cluster of warts in and around the right big toe. Years went by, with the client seeing me every few months or so, and the warts only seemed to be gradually spreading. The client was self-conscious about them, even offering for me to use gloves when conducting the session if needed, so bringing up their meaning would inappropriately stress the relaxing session.

Then, out of the blue and without saying a word, the warts completely vanished. No treatment was sought; they just independently disappeared of their own accord. Witnessing this phenomenon after years of working with this client, I had to ask the deeper questions. They relayed that major closure had just been afforded to them through a recent passing in the family, which released long held tensions; they felt their mind was at peace for the first time in a very long time. This was a perfect meaning for the wart's sudden disappearing act.

My second story is more of a rarity, but I cannot deny that it makes for a good book. I had a client that presented me with a very large wart on their ball of the left foot in Vertical Zone Three. The wart was so distinct and so gnarly that I could not deny the malicious intent of the marker in that area. Post-session, I relayed my findings and questioned the client pointedly about the state of their left lung. Having passed the test, my client revealed to me that indeed they had found a mass in the left lung and that they were scheduled to have it removed in two weeks. Since then, we now monitor the wart's state. It has gone through many healing changes since the surgery; developing a hole at one stage, callousing over in another and now being sucked back into the body gradually.

There is an underlying theme of work related emotional tensions that accompany a marker like this. As our sessions progress, educating a client like this on both sides of the marker's story have been very beneficial. To be clear, not every wart means a malicious growth of tissue and I have only seen one true case of this so far. However, should a marker seem suspicious there is no harm is getting it checked out by a physician. This client and I had an established rapport; I would not have been so direct to a new client that I just met and there would have been a very different use of words. Always exercise caution and use common sense when assessing dramatic markers.

Air

Light, Thin and Circulatory

There is a healthy contrast to follow our discussion of Earth and its symptomology with Air and its opposite characteristics. While Earth is stable, Air is mobile. While Earth is predicable, Air is ever sporadic. While Earth creates structure and systems, Air rushes about freely. The two remind each other of what it is to be in balance. Earth reminds Air to have a schedule or it will be late. Air reminds Earth to not be so hard headed. Earth reminds Air to be diligent in one's efforts. Air reminds Earth to pick up the pace because getting it done is better than getting it perfect.

A case can be made for each element's value. Ultimately, there must be a balance. One cannot exist without the other and the fierce contrast of these two forces being out of balance within the body is easy to see. As with Earth, each element has a unique physical trait. Air's trait is being physically narrow or ***Thin***. Thinness, as opposed to width, indicates an overall lack of resources. Having too much in your possession ties you down and Air is all about being free. Injecting the image of a bird here is very appropriate as people with an Air constitution often eat and live in a birdlike fashion: flitting from place to place in their own little world, picking up an insect or berry here or there, and always on the move.

Additional traits for Air include a more pallid complexion with fairer skin and hypermobility of the joints. Earth's solidness and lack of swift circulation lend to a denser complexion, while Air's flighty and rapid metabolism leave the skin almost bleached in color. Likewise, the tough and strong ligaments that go along with the dense bones of Earth's structure cannot be found in Air. Air's ligaments are loose and hypermobile, meaning that when you go to move the tissues of the foot there will be an effortless over-extension past normal alignment.

Air's signature markers include dryness and lines within the tissues. Different from palmistry, there are no fixed lines on the feet and we do not assess lines that are present in an oracular fashion. Instead, lining and fissures in the feet represent a lack in vital nutrients and that the tissues have become so weak they are beginning to split.

Patches of dryness within the feet are often dismissed, but I find them to be a universal sign of exhaustion. Dryness occurs from the body withdrawing circulation, where that occurs in the reflexes provides the Reflexologist with a direct map of where someone is feeling drained physically, mentally and emotionally.

With all of that information in mind, let's bounce into Air symptomology:

Common Air Symptomology by Zone

Horizontal Zone One

<u>Narrow Toes</u> — We discussed wide toes in the previous section, but narrow being the mark of Air brings the opposite qualities. Thin toes represent a thin and more mobile head/neck space, which can also be overly mobile. An internal component of narrow toes is a narrow mental focus. Not necessarily a limited mind, as Air is quite sharp intellectually, but more a limited attention time to objects of desire. This narrow focus is fully present, but only lasting a short while as opposed to the widened and sustained perspective of Earth.

<u>Space Between Toes</u> — Seemingly benign, but simple spacing between specific toes can indicate powerful information in relation to one's thoughts and how the Vertical Zones are playing together. When space is present between the toes, there is a disconnect between those two Vertical Zones both physically and internally. Taking each toe's meaning into account is very important here.

<u>Dry Toes</u> — As already mentioned, dryness in all its forms indicated levels of exhaustion due to over circulation. The body has begun to withdraw vital resources from the tissues in question. The toes are the reflexes for the head and neck, so the dryness invading this area of the foot paints the picture of exhausted nature of the eyes, sinuses, neck and head. Internally, the mind is spent and the one's mental energy has been

expended to such a degree that the natural balance has shifted towards showing an empty tank.

Hypermobile Toes – The denseness of ligaments is not present within a hypermobile body. When we apply this looseness to the head and neck, we see tendencies for headaches due to the cervical vertebrae constantly shifting in and out of place. From a softer angle, the individual hypermobile toe is significant in relation to the Vertical Zone on which this marker is present; some toes will be more flexible than others. These loose toes show us a lack of solid opinions in relation to that Vertical Zone and over-flexible thoughts that are hard to nail down. Building your library of experience by palpating multiple toes will provide you a gauge for what constitutes a loose or stiff toe.

Deep Creases – Lining differs in severity. However, wherever lining is present the tissues are drying out due to excess Air circulation; not in terms of physical air, but the elemental traits of running around past your limits without proper scheduling and the lack of grounding routines such as meals, self-care and the like. Creases on the tops of the toes represent a fatigued neck. The feet will also show this symptom as an overtaxed mind that literally begins to halt proper word formation due to its fatigue. Sometimes, the lines are vertical and under the toes, the line orientation normally does not mean anything to me but the lines being under the toes would move those meanings directly into the throat reflex area.

Cracked Toe Skin - A very distinguishable and visible marker to be sure; splits are truly a great divide in the tissues on all accounts. When a fissure or deep crack surfaces on a toe there is a sign of deep weakness in the physical and mental/emotional aspect of that reflex area. The rift can be physically in the head/neck or it can be an exhaustion of one's capacity to vocalize what is on their mind in relation to that Vertical Zone.

Split Toenails – Although common, this marker is a powerful signal from the body that needs to be delicately handled. Many clients have argued with me about injury causing this marker, but I tell you from personal experience (*and based on coaching tools I will teach you later in this book about how to develop a proper timeline*) that the meaning of this marker is always relevant and never something to be brushed off. A fractured toenail is a fractured mind; that's the brunt of it. The mental state has come to a very clear split, the larger the split the greater the internal division. Physically, there is degeneration within the soft tissues of the face, but I find in my experience that the internal marker takes precedence.

Split Toenail Story: A business colleague of mine once came in for a Reflexology session with the intention of relieving their foot pain. They knew of my skills with assessment and apologized for their feet in advanced, but there was no way to prepare for the conversation we would have post-session. Immediately spotting a massive split on the left big toe and several smaller splits scattered throughout Horizontal Zone One, I got the inkling that we were going to have some therapeutic dialogue after their time on the table. Migrating back out to my front desk area, with no one else around, we began to discuss the split in the left big toe nail. "Oh yeah, that happened a long time ago. I was about nineteen when I dropped a heavy tool right on the toe and the toe just never healed."

This was very surprising to me as normally the body chooses to heal fractures, but not in this case. So I explained the significance of such a split and questioned my colleague regarding if they felt their mental state was represented by the meaning of this nail. Some tears were had and the conclusion was that there was a great divide in their mind about how to move forward in life. It seemed that every time my colleague followed their passion, they ended up broke and worse for it. Then, they would enter the corporate dynamic, business a reputable company and become terribly depressed because they were making money but had lost their enthusiasm for life; the cycle would then repeat.

Within a situation such as this one, there is a tenderness that must be applied generously. Suggestions are made from a place of compassion and meanings given in a textbook and inquisitive tone rather than an accusatory one. At the end of our discussion the advice I gave my colleague was to let their symptoms be their guide. Obviously, the mental split was still present after all these years. By applying self-care and reading up on the content of other business owners who have lived through the same dilemma, there would be a gradual repair of the nail as the body and mind came to together. Giving the awareness and power back over to the individual is the goal of this coaching; they were now fully equipped and engaged to conquer a long-held issue that the feet had clearly vocalized for some time.

Lack of Toenail – If a split nail represents a fracture of the soft tissues within the face, a missing nail is a complete recession of those tissues. This can be an indicator of sinus, eye and dental problems. Another internally significant marker, the nail literally is the structure that protects the toe; just like the mind develops patterns and thought processes to function in daily life. When a nail is missing, those contextual thought patterns have left the building and the mind becomes impressionably delicate. A word of advice to those struggling with or have friends/family/clients with a missing nail, know this marker and its meaning well. Nails can grow back and if they do it means a restoration of those mental faculties, but as the nail continues to be absent you should always err on the side of caution when in discussions as the mind's defenses are perpetually down.

Horizontal Zone Two

Lack of Tissue – Interesting to find as this is not the norm, but some people just have less padding on the balls of the feet. Similar to our discussion about width in this area, we are discussing the physical reflexes of the chest/lungs/shoulders and the internal feelings/emotions of that individual. Less tissue means less tissue, it is a literal meaning. This individual will be prone to having weak chest and shoulder muscles, and also a lesser capacity for emotions. People with certain thinness in any zone will be less strong in that zone on all levels; here we apply that to the chest area and the emotional state.

Lines on the Ball – Lining is commonly confused as scarring because of how precise and deep the lining can be on the ball of the foot - normally consisting of a single, well-defined line that runs vertically from the Shoulderline Guideline to the Diaphragm Guideline. The Air here has created a collapsing tendency within the chest complex that could be related to any physical reflex in the zone. Emotionally, it does represent the feeling of being scarred. The line's direct location in line with a specific toe can change the meaning based on the Vertical Zone as we get into deeper story building.

Split Skin – Sometimes common callousing on the ball of the foot can become so dry and dehydrated that it splits. Here we learn to combine Earth and Air in meaning based on what elemental markers you see present. The split skin, as a representation of Air, is the fissure of weakness over the physical reflexes where the splitting has occurred. Emotionally, there can be an interesting blending of meaning, but the marker itself is the Air scarring that occurs from long periods of emotional exhaustion that results in the metaphorical heart feeling separated.

Plantar Wart – It begs to be mentioned here that a true plantar wart is most commonly found in the ball of the foot. This is a sign of a literal hole in the heart as a true plantar wart resembles a small black hole in the tissue. Again, a plantar wart is different from a regular wart because a regular wart is an external growth and a plantar wart is an internally focused pit. Although this marker can be read physically, I find the mental/emotional significance powerful enough.

Plantar Wart Story: After a presentation I gave on Reflexology, a woman came up to me from the audience who had a question for me. She was visibly not well and I knew there was much more to the story than physical wellness. The woman proceeded to slip off her left shoe and show me a plantar wart in Horizontal Zone Two and Vertical Zone Two. She said that this wart had been there for two months and nothing she was doing had worked to get rid of the thing. I was visibly struck by the placement of the wart so central in two and two; she must have seen this on my face.

I slowly relayed in a softer tone that this was a very emotional marker that was similar in meaning to a hole in the heart. Taking a brief pause, I continued to explain that the timeframe of the plantar wart's arrival was very significant and the duration of the water would be directly related to the duration of the emotional turmoil that was currently being experienced. With no visible emotion, with the same look on her face, the woman bluntly stated that her mother had passed two months ago and that my interpretation made sense.

With another quick and somewhat frustrated tone, the woman questioned if there was indeed anything to be done about the wart. I again confirmed that nothing could be done until the emotions had been released. Being satisfied with my echoed answer, she put her sock and shoe back on and left. The emotional weight surrounding the interaction was physically palpable, but the woman was so strong that she did not open an inch during our conversation. No wonder the body had manifested the symptom. It was a physical reminder of what she had yet to deal with.

Horizontal Zone Three

<u>Pits</u> – Now, you can find pitting anywhere in the foot, but I do find it most commonly in Horizontal Zone Three. Pitting refers to a visual or textural lack of tissue that forms a pocket within a certain area. If you were walking over a reflex with Reflexology technique you would feel a sudden drop under your pressure. Visually, there can be sudden dips or holes (*not actual holes, but noticeable areas of different substance*) in the tissues as well. Because Air is light and lacks heaviness, pitting regularly indicates weakness or lack of strength in the tissues. Being related to the upper digestive area, accounting for the different reflexes present on

each foot, pitting here indicates emptiness or lacking in this center. The liver should be dense, flush and feel spongey, and should not contain pits of weakness. Even the stomach being hollow, should not have pits of weakness which may indicate a lack of nutrient intake.

Mentally/Emotionally, Horizontal Zone Three is the center of our career and actions. Finding weakness or over-flexibility here can mean a variety of things, ranging from being lethargic in one's duties to a lack of structured scheduling when tackling daily tasks. Although I do see a more overly-aggressive and fiery flavor to the zone, when Air is present the natural upper digestive fires have burnt out and are not performing up to par. Likewise, the drive, passions and enthusiasm normally contained within Horizontal Zone Three has become fatigued.

Fatigued Kidneys – Technically the kidney reflexes straddle Horizontal Zone Three and Four, but we will mention them here. Seeing dry, lined or pitted kidney reflexes are a quick and easy marker to spot. When you see a small bean-shaped patch of dryness, concentrated lines and/or pitting in the center of the sole of the foot there is fatigue in the kidney reflex area. The mental/emotional marker can be considered, but I find this particular issue to have a stronger physical interpretation.

Peeling – When tissues choose to release, they can often release in very fun and visually impressive ways. Peeling is the central marker for this releasing or shedding process; embodying a new found freedom and a fresh layer of self emerging. Physical tissues are being released in the area associated with this marker. I see this most often during digestive duress or after something like a colonoscopy, where internal shedding has occurred in the upper GI tract. Internally, when peeling occurs in this zone there is a career and actions transition, often associated with a change in direction that redefines one's orientation of productivity. When peeling occurs once there is a wonderful sense of release. However, when there is constant peeling over and over without end, then there is a feeling of the body and mind seeking to purge something that is for whatever reason not easy to let go of.

Peeling Feet Story: One day, I received an email from a regular client of mine expressing reservations about booking their next appointment. They had developed an outbreak of peeling skin on the soles of their feet and wondered whether it was appropriate to come and see me in this condition. I have known this client for years; I know their family and their lifestyle, none of which was conducive to contracting a skin fungus. I encouraged the client to schedule a session anyways and if it was truly something of concern then we just wouldn't conduct the hands-on work. Upon arrival, I took a peek at the client's feet before proceeding with our session. Sure enough, there were two patches of peeling skin smack dab in the center of Horizontal Zone Three and Vertical Zones Three and Four on both feet.

My questioning began and I medically went down the checklist of potential infections, but there were no signs of Athlete's Foot or other contagions. So, I began to ask more pointed questions about career stress, to which my client's face promptly lit up. They began to relay an elaborate series of events that had taken place over the past three weeks beginning with my client meeting with their long-term employer to hand in their resignation. After the meeting my client erupted in a shingles outbreak that wrapped around their upper core (*also Horizontal Zone Three*). At the same time, the skin on the soles of their feet began to shed and it was now dying down, but still noticeably present.

Bringing all of this into perspective, my client's body was releasing massive amounts of energy from their nervous system. Despite wanting to leave their job, there was more attachment than even they realized and the entire situation was emotionally super charged. The suggestion I gave was to not get sucked into the void created by the new found freedom (*Air*) post-employment. Instead, creating a solid structure (*Earth*) to channel their energies into productive activities is needed for the body, mind and spirit to refocus into the next venture.

Horizontal Zone Four

<u>Bleached Skin</u> – What I am referring to here is, compared to the other tissues of the feet, the soles seem to be very pale. I call this being 'bleached' because it looks as if the skin as been exposed to a lightening agent, when in fact it is another way the body reveals Air in the tissues. When I see bleaching of any kind, although most common holistically or locally in the digestive reflexes, there is a theme of malnutrition and lack of energy. When the digestive reflexes take on this color change it means that those organ reflexes are delicate, flighty and often sporadic in their duties. Food sensitivities are common symptoms and anemic tendencies as well. Internally, there is weakness of purpose and relational support.

<u>Collapsed Arch</u> – Earth gives us an overview of the importance of arch structure, but let's zoom in on the significance of a collapsed arch. What I define as a collapsed arch is an arch that, when the person is standing, does not lift from the ground and instead lies flat. Standing is the only real way to measure arch height because a faux arch can masquerade as a fully formed arch if the person's feet are lifted from the ground. The arch itself must contain an appropriate amount of ligament rigidity and muscular tension to be held to form, but a fallen arch is not a purely bad thing. Many people I know survive wonderfully with a flat arch. There are some physical and internal predispositions that need to be understood, but a collapsed arch is not necessarily bad, it's just a constitutional difference.

Flatter feet occur due to two primary factors; here we will be discussing hypermobility of the ligaments (Air), but there is also a lack of muscular tone (Fire) that contributes as well. Having an arch with this looseness gives looseness to the spine, making the bones easy to self-adjust in and out of place – for better or worse. There is also a loosened and weak digestive system that can be prone to constipation due to lack of Horizontal Zone Four integrity. A person with super flexible and airy Horizontal Zone Four tissues has an open and free association to family and relationships, often recharging their personal energies through interactions with others and having a less structured definition within that sphere of one's life.

Ankle Hypermobility – While the arch represents the spine, the ankle represents the hip complex with the medial ankle being more in the midline of the pelvis and the lateral ankle being the outer edge of the pelvis. Having a hypermobile ankle brings physical instability and over-flexibility to the hips. The ankle feels like it's made of rubber in this case or that the bones are constantly shifting in and out of place. We can apply the same internal meaning to a hypermobile arch, but the underlying theme here is a lack of solid support. If the relationships of the bones don't stack appropriately to provide alignment, then there is an internal equivalent of feeling that their inner circle is lacking that support.

Reproductive Story: One of the things I see the most in my practice are women who have a common blend of symptoms that tailspin into a health crisis. Normally, we will start by trying to manage their headaches or migraines, but there is always the same trifecta of underlying issues present; I see that the headaches/migraines at the tip of a much larger iceberg. This trifecta of issues is a combination of reproductive weakness, anxiety and digestive distress. We will discuss anxiety and digestive distress heavily in the Fire and Water element sections, but reproductive weakness is a 100% Air condition. The marker here is simple; the ligaments of the dorsal ankle (*where the foot turns into the shin*) become weak and distended, so much so that the foot falls forward. This looseness takes place right over the fallopian tube reflexes and represents a physical collapse in the reproductive system.

The goal with situations like these is to understand the balance of elements that are contributing to the weakness in the reproductive reflexes. There is Air in the reproductive system that is indicative of hormonal imbalance. Taking into consideration other elements present within the reflexes and cross-referencing them with the clients' feedback is the next step. This is how we create the story, to be fully expanded upon later, but it all boils down to bringing balance to the elements present. From there we are able to unwind the symptom at the tip of the iceberg by chipping away at the contributing factors.

Although not always the case, but normally seventy percent of the time, there is a common thread of eating dis-orders within clients of this symptomology. We counterbalance Air with Earth by bringing nutrients to the weakened tissues through regularly planned meals that are filled with substance. Increasing calorie intake with truly rich food containing lots of vegetables and proteins can be an easy fix to a dramatic series of health inconsistencies. Clients have reported immediate relief from the headaches/migraines, digestive distress, anxiety and reproductive symptoms that accompany a body that is asking for such substance and regularity.

Horizontal Zone Five

<u>Thin Heels</u> – Heels are not always large and padded. Sometimes a client will have heels that are the smallest part of their entire foot – this is very significant to how the body and the person are distributing their energies. A narrowness in the heels means a lack of substance in the lower body reflexes leading to weak knees, potential for sciatica and less energy in that zone. Horizontal Zone Five is the home of our sense of security and how we are moving forward, so having less physicality in this zone represents a tendency to not put down roots, move from place to place and have an overall more carefree approach to life.

<u>Dry Heels</u> – The withdraw of vital fluid and nutrients from the heels indicates a starving lower body and sense of security. Exhaustion has drained the structures of the legs and fatigue has infiltrated the process of moving forward. Varying degrees can be present ranging from patches of dryness to full on white across the entire surface. The progression or recession of this symptom is based on the level of stability one cultivates towards a rooted foundation.

Cracked Heels – Splitting heels is a major concern for many people. They can't wear sandals, potentially painful and the sharp nature of the cracks can sometimes hurt others that are close (*having worked on plenty of feet with these cracks, I know their pain all too well*). The general consensus of my clients is that no amount of creams, balms or lotions can help. I tend to agree, because the issue is internal. I will literally call this marker 'cracks in the foundation' because there is a very real physical and mental/emotional equivalent to that statement. Repairing such cracks requires a mending of the Earth element through scheduled self-care and getting back to the basic necessities of life. Air is the element of sporadic over-exertion. Yes, we can nicely say that it is also about freedom, expansion and swiftly achieving one's goals, but if chronic cracking is in your heels, it's time to buckle down and get back to a regular predicable routine ASAP.

Fire
Colorful, Long and Hot

We are warned against playing with Fire. Thankfully for you and this book, I ignored the warning and have gained a vital understanding of how Fire behaves. I am no arsonist, but I do consider myself a firefighter of sorts. I have seen this element in its full glory as it engulfs certain reflexes and reduces various body systems to cinders. Naturally, there is always a balance and I have met quite a few remarkable individuals who have learned to partner with the Fire in their constitution – being fully aware of Fire's dangers and advantages.

The first and most obvious trait of Fire is its brightness and color since light is perceived faster than heat. For this reason, Fire within the reflexes will be most obviously spotted by its flamboyant shades of red. Redness, in various hues, is an indicator of the dramatic dilation vasculature. With that increased circulation brings heat, pressure and redness. Where this redness takes place is extremely significant as it is a literal red flag of inflamed areas within the body's reflexes. That being said, another red flag, that may or may not be visibly red, indicating Fire's presence will be reflex areas that are hot to the touch. Learning to

FOOT READING

decode these heightened areas on the feet is an easy and essential skill to develop for the aspiring Foot Reader.

Air and Fire are very similar in their indication of movement, but Fire differs from Air due to its dependent nature. Fire as an element requires a fuel source and is largely limited to the surrounding area of that fuel source. This fact makes for an interesting dynamic of where Fire chooses to appear in the body. Just like in nature, fires occur in dried out areas that were once plant rich (*Earth*), but have withered (*Air*) to produce perfect kindling. The missing element is a spark, a perfect reference to a stressor if there ever was one, including physical trauma, mental disturbance and/or emotional upheaval – the tipping point for a deprived individual to erupt into various stages of pyrotechnics.

Some people just run hot though and the Fire foot is visibly characterized by its **Length**. Lewd references aside, Fire feet are assertive, charismatic and somewhat invasive. Another characteristic of the Fire constitution is its athletic musculature, often too tight, that is visible through the dynamic array of tendons and arch support present in the Fire foot. As a final touch, we can always see a Fire foot garnished with visible redness as if to warn a passersby of the fervent nature this foot's owner possesses. Just like their feet, people holding great Fire in their constitutions will make their presence known through a variety of spirited twists and turns; nothing can be as entertaining as working with a Fire foot.

Common Fire Symptomology by Zone

Horizontal Zone One

Longer Toes – A fascinating phenomenon is the subject of toe length. If you haven't seen the genealogy meme relating toe length to cultural ancestry, you've been living under a rock. Toe length does not indicate family history, but it does show someone's distribution of energy across the five Vertical Zones in Horizontal Zone One i.e. what they think about most and what areas of their life they have the most energetic resources. Long toes indicate a fierier headspace and longer head/neck reflexes, but the real value for this marker is in length discrepancy. Pay attention to toe length if you want to know the ins and outs of what is most important to that person.

Hot Toes – When I first began to discover the world of listening to what the feet had to say, one of the most astounding things for me was to feel how certain toes would be hot, like really hot to the touch. This was even before I cracked the code on elemental assessment, so the weirdness of this marker for me was confounding. Heat in the toes is equivalent to heat in the head, whether through pressure, injury or inflammation – the Fire is in the headspace for some reason and your goal should be to figure out why. Because Fire is associated with charged feelings of general excitement, I have found that redness and heat doesn't always mean 'turning red with anger'. However, the internal meaning of red toes does indicate a fire in the mind, which could range from excitement and general over activity to the classic intense anger.

Flushing from White to Red – Interesting to see, but not a healthy marker overall. Bleaching of the tissues in any case is an Air marker, a sign of more fragile constitution. When pressure is applied to toes that seem pallid, you will sometimes see a prominent flash of red circulation. The message here is that the tissues of the head and face, upon receiving stress, become quickly inflamed. Internally, when the mind is put under duress there is a dramatic and excited reaction. Continuing to trend in the direction of interesting, flashy toes like this may or may not return to their normal color right away. Noticing how long it takes for the toe color to reset also factors into the meaning.

Gout – Another favorite of mine. Normally, Gout is known as the King's Disease and is medically diagnosed as a buildup of acidic crystals within the big toe joint. Allow me to deviate from this interpretation and to relay my experience seeing clients with Gout. If a bunion is a bottling up of emotions and a pressure in the chest, then Gout is when the metaphorical heart had been doused in napalm and set ablaze due to the amount of stress one is under.

Curiously, there is variation as to where the heat lands in a Gout case. Sometimes the heat is in the toe pad, other times it's in the neck of the toe, while it can also be present in the bunion area itself. Physically, there is massive heated restriction, spasm and pain in the corresponding reflex area. All indicate a different interpretation based on location, but the symptom's internal meaning is the same: intense rage that is so inflammatory it cannot be suppressed any longer.

Horizontal Zone Two

Heat in the Heart – The ball of the foot is both the physical and emotional heart center of the feet. I regularly see this area having excess heat on the plantar surface when there is a building of inflammation and over-excited emotions in the chest. Often paired with the Water marker of fluid retention, a hot ball of the foot by itself definitely indicates that any physical symptom will be heart/lung related and will have a strong emotional component attached.

Morton's Neuroma – When this diagnosis is given, there is reference to nerve pain in the ball of the foot. However, the cause is always emotional in my experience. Neuromas will mysteriously come and go based on internal stress, above any other cause. There is a correlation with shoulder entrapment and rotator cuff issues, but I find that painful emotions are the root of this specific symptom.

Inflamed Bunions – We discussed bunions already as part of the Earth markers, indicating structural deviation and pressure within the center of the chest. Some bunions have a stronger Fire component than others. When you add in the Fire element to an already deviated bunion, there will be added pain and emotional excitement in its meaning. I will often find a single red (Fire) and swollen (Water) bunion (Earth) on the left side as a trifecta marker indicating a true heart condition. However, emotionally there are grades of agitation when considering how hot, red and painful a bunion is overall.

Popped Tendons – Ligaments and bones are the property of Earth, but tendons and muscles are related to Fire as the combustion engines and movers of the body. When tendons pop anywhere in the feet, there is an increase in muscular tension present in those reflex areas. Internally, there is an over-driven tendency within that mental/emotional zone. I often see popped tendons on the dorsal aspect of the foot in Horizontal Zone Two, indicating tight upper back muscles and surface emotional tension that just won't quit. Be sure to notice the Vertical Zone(s) where tendons pop and practice your gridding wisely.

Gas Pedal Foot – This is one of the easiest markers to identify when seeing a new client once you build your rolodex by seeing this foot shape. As a client relaxes their feet for you to read (*not planted on the ground, but preferably elevated on a massage table or reclining chair*) you will notice that there is a distinctive shape that forms in people who have an excess of Fire in their system: it looks as if their foot is always on the gas pedal of a car. This is due to the ball of the foot being pushed forward, which is often red and puffy as well due to excess emotional stress. When this marker is present it is another sign of fiery feelings and also inflammation in the chest cavity. These clients will also have trouble relaxing as they are always on the go-go-go.

Horizontal Zone Three

Gas Pedal Foot Continued – Now, there is a dual-action happening with a Gas Pedal Foot. In order for the ball of the foot to jut forward the soft tissues of the metatarsals in Horizontal Zone Three must physically become contracted and tightened. Sometimes, there will only be tension in Horizontal Zone Two, or just in Three, so let's go over the second meaning – the difference can be felt through basic palpation. If Horizontal Zone Three is contracted, hot and red with Fire, then the upper digestive reflexes are very much affected.

Yes, the stomach, spleen, liver and gallbladder are the workhorses that help to filter and process our system through the heat of metabolism, but this marker indicates that the person is working too hard and there is a theme of burning up energy faster than one can consume it. Likewise, the drive to succeed in one's career has become so great that they risk being engulfed by the flames of their own motivation. In both cases, the need to slow down, calm one's self and move forward at an even pace is required for long-term health.

<u>Overheated Stomach Reflex</u> – In the case listed above, I sometimes see that the left foot is affected by Fire while the right is not – let's discuss this. When the stomach/spleen/pancreas reflex area is overheating there is a tendency for acid reflux, ulcers, an obviously upset stomach and an over-production of the digestive hormone and enzymes. Internally, one's current career situation is pushing them too hard and they need to back off. Speaking as someone who personally works with this marker on a regular basis, I can tell you that the feet will begin to glow red, become hot and muscularly tight as I burn the midnight oil too many weeks in a row.

<u>Angry Liver</u> – The liver reflex is on the right foot due to the actual organ being on the right side of the body. When only the right side of Horizontal Zone Three is fired up there is a sign of a liver/gallbladder reflex that have to work way too hard. I will often see diabetics, alcoholics, cleanse-addicts and people who are struggling to process their past actions with this marker. Essentially, the liver and gallbladder, both in form and energetic function, are overheating while trying to process and transmute the items being funneled to them.

Hot Kidney Story: As the story goes, "There once was a man from out of state, whose kidneys were truly irate. He came to see me for a foot rub you see, but left having learned his fate."

Every so often I get a true health scare that I see through the reflexes. This man had come to see me because he got Reflexology wherever he traveled for work and he traveled A LOT. He loved my approach to the work, relaxing and subtle, paired with specific point work to move congestion out of the body through the nerves in the feet. However, I did not expect to find what I did.

In a bean-shaped formation, perfect branded into both feet, were fiery patches of skin. Understanding that this meant excess heat in the kidneys I knew that drinking water would be in our conversation post-session, but these patches were truly on fire and congested – so much so that I had to bring it to his attention in a stronger way. After the hands-on technique, I met him back up at the front desk and proceeded to share how strongly I felt that he needed to be aware of his hydration and kidney area. Upon relaying that message, the client relayed that he had indeed recognized that all the traveling and unhealthy dietary patterns made him feel like he could potentially have a kidney stone forming.

At that moment, having confirmation of my findings and my client's own intuition of his body, I echoed my findings again and warned that if water was not made a priority that the body would raise the volume on the discomfort in the very near future. He appreciated the tone of my voice and stated that it was refreshing to work with a Reflexologist who had the ability to see into the body. I reminded him that the body was trying to tell him what was wrong, but he ignored it and without the body's help I wouldn't have seen the marker – it is the natural intelligence of the body at work, a Reflexologist learning to interpret the message isn't the headline of the story here.

Never again did I see this client, but the story is one I hold as a 'close call' for someone who was truly on the edge of a health crisis.

Horizontal Zone Four

<u>Burnt Out Gut</u> – What will happen when someone struggles with Horizontal Zone Three (*upper digestive and career*) issues for a long period of time is that the Fire will exhaust and burn out the upper Horizontal Zone Three and move down into the more personal Horizontal Zone Four. The tissues of this lower zone slowly start to take on the heat, redness and tension that were previously held in the above zone. Physically, what has begun to happen is the chronic

over-production of digestive acids within the upper GI tract that are now affecting the more sensitive lower GI tract. Internally, we have the career stress starting to trickle into the family environment. This is more dangerous than it sounds internally because the individual has become so exhausted from their activities that they have begun to inflame their innermost relationships. When this occurs, a major priority shift needs to take place.

<u>Heated Pockets</u> – An entire zone may be affected by any one element, but a common marker I see relates to specific sections within that zone holding a concentrated amount of the elemental infection. I see this mostly in Horizontal Zone Four as the organs themselves in the lower core/pelvis are prone to stagnant pocketing. Here we find individual pockets of Fire in the lower GI, or bladder/reproductive depending on location, which are specifically placed to convey symptomology. I'm referencing most 'oil lamp' conditions such as diverticula and digestive lining issues where the tract with stagnate, harden and coagulate fluid, but then acquire an infection or irritation - taking on an oil lamp quality.

<u>Over-Developed Arch</u> – High arches are just arches with greater tension which warps the bones into a new shape. With the muscles literally firing with greater intensity, there is a systemic ripple of the same phenomenon throughout the body as well – the body is just too hot. Specifically, we know Horizontal Zone Four as the main lift in the arch, so there is greatest tension within the reflexes of the low back, hips and pelvic area. What I find interesting about individuals with high arches is that they put very heavy demands on their relationships – always choosing to act independently, then wondering why no one is there to help them.

Let's Talk about High Arches: We need to address this quality because you will find it highly valuable when seeing these types of clients. High arches that are muscularly out of control have two ways to interpret the meaning: 1) The nice way to say it is that these individuals are highly motivated, driven and independent individuals who are able to function well in high pressure situations 2) The not-so-nice way to say it is that high arches indicate someone who is wound so physically and internally tight that they are unable to surrender their stress for fear of losing motivation and momentum i.e. they thrive in stress that they create for themselves.

These interpretations are two sides of the same coin, but both belong to the Fire constitution. When working with these high arched individuals it is important to remind them that their natural need to go-go-go is not a bad thing. Yes, stay out of their way when they are on the war path, but do not feel bad if they are constantly restless, working too hard, taking on unneeded responsibility or focused on twenty different things at once – it's who they are. I liken high arched individuals to sharks in the way that they must stay moving to breathe (*which is a quality they share with Air*).

Most importantly, do not try to unwind the high arch – this is a futile task because you would be disrupting the natural state of their constitution and Fire bodies also don't appreciate being told what to do. You can assist through manual therapies like Reflexology to balance the arch and the connecting body tissues, but just know that people with a Fiery constitution will always have a healthy lean towards tight, muscular and spasmodic tendencies within their bodies.

Horizontal Zone Five

<u>Hot Heels</u> – Again, heat will select where it is present based on which reflex area has the most inflammation. In the case of the heels we have sciatic nerve inflammation as the symptomology. The heat could relay a variety of individual symptoms including leg pain, cramping or spasm. Hot heels also represent someone's need to get moving into a more stable sense of security, which could be a physical move or an internal transition towards a more grounded vantage point.

<u>Plantar Fasciitis (PF)</u> – I have had many clients come to me with PF and if there is one word to describe them all it is *inconsistent*. Some report direct center of the heel pain that is worse in the morning and takes on a stabbing quality; while others point to the outside of the ankle, inside of the arch, all along the bottom of the foot and even into Horizontal Zone Two. The reports are varied, but there is always pain and a mysterious timeline that is unique to each person.

What I have found is that there is an overwhelming sense of the PF sufferer having lost their sense of security and gained the inability to move forward – they are stuck between a rock and a hard place with moving forward presumably outside of their control. From the standpoint of physical symptomology, there is no concrete way to identify what is causing the serious pain other than directly palpating the reflexes. Often there is no evidence in the way of imaging technology. The whole makeup of this condition is nerve based and occurs from an overload of the pressure within the system. Understanding the major components of internal security being compromised is the major factor.

A Note on Pain, Cramping and Spasms…

I have a very firm stance on pain due to my own experiences with it and feeling pain second hand through my clients. Pain always has a message and reason behind it. Fire is the most dramatic of the four elements and will produce the most striking symptoms, with pain being the most crippling. From a Foot Reading perspective, pain equals pain on both a physical and internal interpretation on the reflexes.

Sometimes, my clients will report pain in a reflex before the pain actually occurs in the corresponding area. Other times, pain occurs in both areas simultaneously. Pain is significant to the assessment and should be read independently, but when pain occurs in a body part and there is no sign of direct reflex issue, I am inclined to look elsewhere in the reflexes for the cause – there is always a cause. Here I would check the reflexes for a corresponding area of weakness that needs to be nourished, which has caused an imbalance to shift into the painful area.

Cramping and spasms are different beasts. Cramps are onetime contractures that are intense and debilitating; while spasms are more in line with repeating twitches that never reach the intensity of a full cramp. Both are Fire symptoms and are muscle related, but cramps are singular eruptions of heat while spasms are like bubbling lava. Having seen so many of these cases, the elemental balance simply needs to be shifted within the individual. Surrounding the person both externally and internally with quiet, dark, stable and nourishing attributes is the goal – just like how you would put out a fire.

The Birthmark Effect

Time and time again I see birthmarks on the feet. At first, with client's strong suggestions that the mark(s) have been there since birth and meant nothing, I discarded them as nothing more than a fluke of nature and something to watch for potential skin cancer. As I have grown as a Foot Reader, birthmarks of all shapes have struck me as significant and I have recently over the past few years understood their meaning. As opposed to the raised moles, warts and growths of Earth, birthmarks are more darkened spots that appear in seemingly random places over time. Some clients have had these marks since birth, but I find more commonly that they mysteriously 'pop up' at different stages of life and health.

The darkened spots on the feet are similar to being burned with a cigarette or an electrical wire that has singed the surrounding structures due to dysfunction. When I have questioned clients about the reflex areas where the birthmark is located they always relay that area as being temperamental – sometimes overactive, other times totally inert. The internal characteristics of the marker hold true as well; to be both a place of excess stress and supreme internal weakness, like an Achilles Heel of sorts. The birthmark area is then interpreted as an area of burnout due to being overused and inefficient. It is as if the body is trying to say: *When everything starts to fall apart, this is where I'm going to fall apart first.*

Water
Pale, Short and Cold

Water is the last of our elements and by now we have plenty of contexts to observe a clear vision of how the others compare and contrast. Earth is stable, wide and dense. Air is circulating, narrow and light. Fire is hot, long and colorful. So, Water must be cold, short and pale. When working on specific individuals I have found that when the feet are cool to the touch, shorter or smaller than they seem like they should be and have a more pallid complexion these are the signs of a Water constitution. As a trifecta, these feet belong to people who are naturally deep, sensitive and emotionally driven, which is pertinent to keep in mind when working with these individuals especially if your temperament is different.

Water in the body is cooling and balancing. The fluid systems of the body, mainly the lymphatic and cardiovascular systems, provide disbursement and homeostatic qualities. Refreshing is an adjective often used to describe the life-giving qualities of this element. However, Water in excess will stagnate and produce tricky symptoms including excess pressure in the physical tissues, a feeling of being overwhelmed and anxious, as well as symptoms that constantly release excess fluid from the tissues. Because of this mischievous nature of Water to mimic other symptoms via fluid pressure and instill emotional panic into those with excess Water in their systems, the cooling and balancing qualities should be kept in mind equally with thoughts of how Water can run out of control in the wild.

Although being **Short** is the key visible trait of a Watery constitution, what these feet lack in length they make up for in depth. Water is known for its ability to create expansive depth under its calm surface; people with a Water constitution fit this description on all levels, and they have lots of levels. People with high levels of Water will rarely be the first to speak up and they prefer to blend into the background or accommodate everyone else's desires. Deep, dark, silence is golden to the hyper-sensitive Water constitution because their powerful undercurrents are providing enough internal chatter as it is. This depth can be seen in the skin in the form of pallor, which occurs when the body withdrawals circulation deep into the core during moments of threat or trauma.

With the obvious symptoms of swelling and sweating aside, Water as an element in the body needs high levels of compassion and clear direction to function; otherwise Water can become cold and unreachable. Take into consideration the hyper-sensitive nature of this element and its associated symptoms. We are dealing with a force that normally balances the other elements and assists in accommodating to the needs of the whole, but when out of control can drown the body in an intensity, depth and duration that the other elements can only dream of.

Common Water Symptomology by Zone

Horizontal Zone One

Swollen Toes – Each toe is significant in and of itself; we know this because of the Vertical Zones of Influence. When we have fluid retention of any kind in the feet there is both a physical gathering of fluid and an internal gathering of emotions present within that reflex area. The toes, representing the head and neck space along with the person's thoughts and opinions, are no different. When the toes are collectively swollen it means just that, fluid and emotion have reached a level of excess within Horizontal Zone One. More commonly though I see a single toe that is filled with fluid, which is much more interesting and you would use the foot that marker is present on and the meaning of that Vertical Zone to interpret.

Congested Toe Pads – Another interesting distinction is when only the pads of the toes are retaining water. If the necks of the toes represent the neck reflexes and one's ability to vocalize, then the pads of the toes are the mind itself and the actual head. Congested toe pads are common in people who present sinus issues, allergies and general pressure in the face; this pressure may manifest in a variety of ways including, but not limited to, eye pressure and dental swelling. Likewise, the mental state would be taking on water which would result in an ocean of thoughts that have amassed a great amount of internal pressure.

<u>Cold Toes</u> – As opposed to Fire, Water brings coolness. An excess of Water in the tissues will chill the reflexes to the bone and produce a clammy texture. When all toes have gone icy there is a deep anxiety or paralyzing fear in the mind; paying attention to the Vertical Zones in the case of a specific toe demonstrating coldness. What this coldness indicates physically is stagnant fluid that needs to be moved and literally warmed up.

<u>Darkened Toe Nails</u> – There are several reasons why a nail can darken, but this darkness brings up several specific issues along with its general meaning. The nails represent the soft tissues of the face and the screen of someone's mind. When darkening of a nail occurs, there is physical stagnation and congestion present and a mental/emotional dark cloud hanging over their head. This meaning stands true regardless of how the darkness manifested, but let's drill down into more specific meanings to better illustrate this marker.

Injury is the first and most common reason why nails will darken and this is due to coagulated blood (Water) under the nail just like what would happen with any other blunt force trauma injury i.e. it's a bruise. Later in this book we will talk about using the adjectives a client selects during a Foot Reading consultation, but it is important to bring up this topic now superficially. Listening to the way a client describes how the injury happens, how long it lasts and/or the sensations present will aide in your assessment. Use the exact wording a client chooses on top of the physical and mental/emotional meaning to better understand the injured nail's significance.

Fungus is a commonly mis-assessed condition. Most individuals who see opaqueness and a rising of their nail's height which they determine as a nail fungus, when really those symptoms are a densifying and growing (Earth) of the nail due to rigidity and not a true fungus. I place nail fungus in the Water category of symptoms because there is a dark, dreary and stagnant appearance to a true nail fungus. The interpretation of such a fungus can be seen as more of an opportunistic infection of the tissues due to lingering long-term stress. The mental state of an individual with standing fungal infections also has a mind that is or has been infected by thoughts that are deep, anxious and are unprocessed.

Random darkening can also occur. In this case, the person has woken up and noticed that one or multiple nails have gone dark, but they cannot figure out the cause. The reason for the darkening may not be known, but the marker is still very present and should be analyzed to figure out the underlying meaning.

Toe Nail Fungus Clients: A have a few clients with fungus under their toe nails. Every time they come in for a session the fungus is the first marker I look at. Over time, I've noticed that when the black finger-like branches of the infection become darker, larger and more pronounced there is a corresponding increase in their reported mental stress and their perspective of situations being out of control. In contrast, when the fungus was noticeably less than normal my clients have a much more positive and balanced view of their current situation. This trend has been surprisingly accurate and I now use it as a gauge for all of my clients with this marker.

Horizontal Zone Two

Puffy Balls of the Feet – Swelling does not always happen universally throughout the feet. There are pockets that can form, just like with the other elemental symptoms, that can be gridded individually; swelling is the same way. Swelling or congestion in the balls of the feet represents fluid buildup in the chest/lung reflex area. Also, an influx of heavy emotions is running amuck, but in contrast to our next marker, puffiness only in the balls of the feet represents internal feelings that are not viewable on the surface. I will often have clients report a lung infection or chest cold when I inquire about feeling of congestion via palpation in the chest/lung reflex area during a Reflexology session.

Dorsal Swelling – When you see a puffiness developing on the topside of Horizontal Zone Two only, this means that the upper back reflexes and lymphatic drainage reflexes have begun to take on excess fluid pressure. The internal equivalent is an emotional surplus that everyone is able to see on the sleeves of that person – very interesting if only one side is presenting the marker as well.

Hair on the Feet – The reason why I am bringing up this marker again is because the Earth marker of hair is often protecting a more sensitive Water constitution. Hair's presence on the tops of the feet, where the hair starts and stops can be mapped on a case by case basis, is extremely telling because the feet have decided the area in question is too sensitive to function without protection. You may think that once hair is present on the feet it stays present – not always. Be aware of where the hair rests and you will find the most emotionally sensitive part of the person you are assessing.

Sweating – During a Reflexology session I will often notice a release of fluid from the feet in Horizontal Zone Two while I work those reflexes. When this happens there is a release of emotions and fluid pressure from the reflexes. I take this as a very good sign and I welcome this marker during any of the work that I do.

Horizontal Zone Three

Puffy Spleen Reflex – I see this particular marker often and its meaning can be applied to any individual reflex, but this is the most common occurrence I've seen. The spleen reflex is located on the left foot in Horizontal Zone Three and Vertical Zone 4 & 5. This section will be raised and fluid-filled on occasion due to an over-active spleen reflex. When noticing such a change in the tissues there will be an immune system component present as if the body is fighting an infection. Yes, we can also interpret this marker mentally/emotionally as current career stress being influenced by family/relationships and how someone is moving forward, but I find the physical reflex meaning more pertinent in this case. Again, this meaning can be applied to any swollen reflex area.

Cold Patches – Water brings frigid temperature when the element is in excess. Cold patches occur where the body has withdrawn circulation and taken vital nutrients deeper into the body. When you find a cold patch in the tissues it means that the body's natural circulation in that area has been dampened and needs to be rekindled. In Horizontal Zone Three, this can manifest as liver / gallbladder / stomach / spleen / pancreas reflex dysfunction and a prolonged anxiety about work situations that are freezing the person in their tracks.

Sweating – Yes, we covered this marker, but the meaning here is independently significant. The upper digestive reflexes, specifically the liver reflex, are key de-toxicants within the interconnected network of body systems. When I notice a large concentration of sweating in this zone, I find the body is also trying to sweat out of the physical and internal toxins from this zone. If you have ever taken care of someone when they are detoxing, you notice an overdose of Water qualities (cold, clammy, pale, sweaty, etc.) as they body attempts to release what is no longer serving them. The same case can be made for the marker of sweating in this zone.

Horizontal Zone Four

Swelling Dorsal Ankle – The dorsal ankle is home to the physical structure of the pelvis and the Fallopian Tube/Vas Deferens reflex, in Reflexology theory. When I see swelling here, there is a building of fluid in the pelvic space. Emotions are also running high in the family/relationship dynamic, but the issues are also on the surface for the world to see due to the swelling being on the dorsal surface.

Swelling Medial Ankle – The medial ankles or medial malleoli are home to the core reproductive reflexes: uterus/prostate. Swelling here can indicate a multitude of reproductive symptomology, but all involving more bloating and pressure; the addition of other elements will add to the meaning. Internally, fluid here indicates thoughts about (*Vertical Zone One*) family and relationships (*Horizontal Zone Four*) that are becoming more emotional.

Swelling Lateral Ankle – The lateral ankles or lateral malleoli are the outside ankle bones and they represent the reflexes for more lateral boney structures of the pelvis: the hip joints. Swelling here indicates more of a fluid retention and lymphatic pressure in those joints, which is normally caused by excess stiffness (*Earth*) so watch for multiple elements being present. Also, the ability to move forward (*Vertical Zone Five*) with family and relationships (*Horizontal Zone Four*) has a buildup of emotional energy.

Congested Vasculature – Whenever you see spider veins or congested vascular of any kind there is a stagnation of Water in the tissues. Visibly, there may be a darkened color to the blood channels. Listen to your client's adjectives and your internal thoughts when describing this marker. Does it look deep? Ugly? Not that bad? Painful? Serious? Superficial? Refer them to a specialist if necessary. Congestion indicates congestion in the physical reflexes and also the mental/emotional meaning of that zone. In Horizontal Zone Four we would see stagnant and congested blood flow in the low back, pelvis, lower GI tract and reproductive reflexes. Looking at the symptom from a subtle vantage point, we would see a sense of backed up feelings in the family/relationship area that have nowhere to go.

Sweating – It needs to be said in conjunction with the meaning of sweating in Horizontal Zone Three, that sweating in Horizontal Zone Four of the foot represents a physical detox or release of tension from the reflexes in that zone. Long held family and relationship feelings will also be let go of when this marker presents.

Bulging Low Back Reflexes – A quick and efficient marker to check for is a little bubble of fluid that will appear in the medial arches in

Horizontal Zone Four, sometimes only on one side. This little bubble is the marker I have found to coincide with herniation of the lower back. This marker can be applied to along the entirety of the spinal reflexes along that medial arch, but I find this simple marker the most. However, I need to mention that clients will claim to have a history of lower back herniation without this marker being present. I gently remind them that discs repair when lifestyle is changed and if the marker is not present, then I am inclined to side with the feet. That does not discount their history, but at the time of my assessment the symptom may not be as present.

Massive Swelling Story: This is a good one. Every once and a while I will have a client come into my office who relays a shocking experience where one foot or both feet swell so intensely that they are concerned for their physical wellbeing. The swelling eventually dissipates, but the seemingly random occurrence sticks out in their mind like a sore toe. After such a story is told, I will politely ask when the swelling took place. After a date has been found and context has been established I gently explain that massive spontaneous swelling in the feet only occurs when the body is under a boat-load of emotional stress.

At that moment, the client will become even more amazed and relay the circumstances surrounding the mysterious swelling. Each and every time there has been a major emotional event (*most commonly a family reunion of some sort*) that was indeed very stressful. The exact timing of the swelling happening and the swelling subsiding directly relates to the height of the stress and the subsequent return to balance post-event. For this reason, I always relate spontaneous swelling to a surge of emotional energy that cannot be contained and the body manifests swelling as the symptom to convey its message of discontent.

There are cases I've worked with where the swelling doesn't go down or lasts over a long period of time. This is when a consultation takes on a more coaching role as the client and I work together to decode the reason for the feet holding on to such a concerning symptom. Water is the element of all things feeling-oriented and its presence needs to be respected with great compassion, but a sense of firmness that helps to guide stagnant feelings towards resolution. Working with a mental health professional may be a perfect addition to interpreting the deeper feeling associated with long-term swelling in the feet.

Horizontal Zone Five

Swollen Heels – Excess fluid in the heels can be palpated easily and will feel like the heel bone itself is incased in a watery layer of tissue that your fingers squish into. Because Horizontal Zone Five is the home of all the leg and lower body reflexes, this marker indicates a stagnation of fluid in the lower body, which can manifest as sciatic pressure, knee discomfort, leg swelling and/or leg vein congestion. The internal component of emotions surrounding how one is moving forward can also be very present. Cardiovascular activity to move the fluid from the lower body and to help the person feel productive in their daily life is a good first step towards balance.

Bubbles – Similar to the bulging low back reflexes, there will sometimes be bubbles of fluid under the skin in Horizontal Zone Five as well. Physically, this marker would be more concerning as fluid pockets in the leg reflexes should be observed by a physician. The pocketing of emotions is also not a healthy way to deal with one's sense of security and how to move forward. This marker is a compartmentalization of the fluid/feelings in this zone and should be worked with to flow properly on all levels.

Bursitis – 'Itis' is the medical suffix for inflammation and is a Fire symptom. However, bursas are fluid-filled sacs that cushion and lubricate the major joints of the body. We have a few of these sacs on the foot, most notably in the heel surrounding the Achilles' Tendon. The bursa itself would represent the feelings (Water) contained within Horizontal Zone Five. When Fire hits the bursa it is like boiling the Water inside, causing even more pressure and steam to build until the bursitis would manifest as a swollen, red and hot lump on the back of the heel.

This is a key marker for sciatic conditions, leg pain and lower body inflammation. Pairing the Fire and Water meanings, we now have an emotionally inflamed sense of security. I find this marker in individuals who are so focused on their to-do list that their body literally has to slow them down with pain; their feet say no, but they keep moving forward well past their limits anyways.

A Note on Hyperhidrosis

The condition presents as feet and other extremities that simply cannot stop sweating. The condition itself is thought of as benign, but from a Foot Reader's perspective there is massive information to be gleaned here. Areas of the feet will sometimes sweat individually and that I've already mentioned multiple times, but there is something unique happening when the entire foot is constantly turning on the waterworks. Having seen this condition across the gambit of ages, races and genders, I can confidently say that the common factor is anxiety.

My personal constitution is very watery. In fact, my hands and feet would sweat all the time and it used to be a serious self-confidence killer for me. I also suffered from serious pent-up anxiety at the time and had little to no self-care regiment to release my stored feelings. So, when I became a bodyworker and noticed this trend in others I was uniquely qualified to share my story to help my clients with this particular symptomology.

The body has a couple of notable signs that it produces when under significant stress that apply to what we are talking about. First, there is coldness when the body withdraws circulation during times of stress and trauma. When you exercise, or are scared, or get the flu, coldness is a sign that the body has manipulated your circulation to better equip you to handle what is happening. Second, there is excretion of sweat and odor to both cool the body and repel attackers. Again, during physical activity, fear, or getting sick, the body makes these other two functions to aide your process.

The problem in the case of a long-standing Hyperhidrotic symptomology is the absence of a life-threating stressor, only the perception of being attacked, invaded and the need to fight, freeze or flee. When a client presents with Hyperhidrosis, there needs to be a productive conversation about stress levels and how they are actively taking time to address those deeper patterns. You can think of this particular symptom as an *Infection of Water*. Similar to how a foot would potentially totally lock up (*Earth*), flare up (*Fire*), or collapse (*Air*), the waterlogged foot needs to be brought back into balance from being overthrown by a single elemental energy.

Blended Elements

There are always exceptions to the rule. Although it would be wonderfully simple to classify people in terms of one elemental constitution alone, that is rarely the case and the body is infinitely more complex than that. Instead, the elemental markers and overall constitutional themes are meant to be guidelines to aid in your assessment skills and to help you use commonly recognizable language with your clients. Some clients may very well have one or two dominant elements within their feet and body, but it is important to note that a blend of each of the four elements is always present.

In relation to constitution there may be one or two dominant elements, or even a perfectly balanced foot, but in markers the story is different. When there are blends of elements present within the zones of the feet I call the markers *stacked*. When markers stack and pile on top of each other there is more energy being spent by the body to get your attention and that is not a good thing. A client coming in with pain in an area and no other markers present is one thing, but a client coming in with pain, swelling, flaking skin and joint impingement all in the same area is a gigantic red flag. The intensity of the marker is compounded by the number of elements blending or stacking together.

> ### Section Recap
>
> o **Elemental language helps both clients and Foot Readers** interpret the markers that are present while using easy-to-understand language to communicate symptomology.
> o The four elements use in Foot Reading to describe markers are: **Earth, Air, Fire and Water.**
> o Earth's key words are: **Density, Width and Growth.**
> o Air's key words are: **Light, Thin and Circulatory.**
> o Fire's key words are: **Colorful, Long and Hot.**
> o Water's key words are: **Pale, Short and Cold.**
> o Everyone has all four elements to some degree, but most clients have **one or two core constitutional elements** that are more dominant.

Coaching Through the Feet

After the basic mapping has been learned and the elements of a symptom understood, there comes the moments when it all needs to be put together into a concise package, wrapped in a pretty bow and presented to the client. This is the art of coaching a client via the markers you find in the feet. I will do my best in this section to explain in detail my science to this process, but it is an art. There are concrete aspects of every dialogue I have in regards to aspects like the timeline, adjectives used and communicating the information I am seeing into a digestible message. At the end of the day there is practice, time and experience that will be the gateway to mastering this advanced aspect of Foot Reading.

When I studied Reflexology I was told that it was a hands-on technique. Studying massage therapy before that conveyed the same message: You must be in the room, doing the technique, in order to succeed. When I began to accrue clients in other states and around the world looking for me to read their feet through the screen of a computer, my conception of what Reflexology and bodywork is and isn't, was flipped on its head – and there was no recovering. The dramatic transformations, testimonials and outpouring of gratitude that came from simply relaying the messages I found in people's feet was an unshakeable reality. It just so happened that there was no hands-on technique involved.

Detaching from the normal definitions of Reflexology and into the realm of Foot Reading has illuminated the theories I have shared in this work. Putting them together for each individual client in a coaching format is a valid way to practice this information, but the hands-on work does help jumpstart the process. I would not be here today without my Reflexology sessions and I certainly would not have been exposed to the same amount of feet without first pursuing the bodywork aspect of this craft. That being said, the two can exist independently of each other, but there is a certain natural magic when they are paired.

I encourage you to delve as deep into the practice of seeing the entirety of the individual through the lens of the feet as you see fit. One side of the coin may call to you more than the other. For me, with my gentler touch, stronger verbal skills and a pointed intuition, assessment has been where I shine (*and likewise the teaching of that assessment*). You voice must be fully expressed through your chosen modality and you may wish to be more hands-on or more dialogue based with your clientele. I have sessions that are solely (*that was a pun*) coaching, either through video or in person, and some that are strictly hands-on. Some hands-on sessions will drift to incorporate more coaching and vice versa as the client and I interact during our time together, but the exchange is organic and always what is needed.

Do not feel that you are more or less noble if you do not incorporate coaching sessions into your practice. Trying to force a verbal exchange that is not within your natural strengths can be awkward for both parties involved. Do not let a discomfort deter you either; many successful endeavors are first approached with hesitancy. Instead, play and seek to find the perfect balance for you as a practitioner. I believe the feet will take you where you need to go. Let them speak to you in the way only they can and everything will work itself out. That's my round-about hippie statement of saying: *Just do the work.*

Putting it all Together

Time and experience is the way you perfect your craft of giving meaning to the markers you find within the feet in a clear and concise manner. There is no substitute for that. The process revolves around developing that rolodex of feet in your mind and gradually seeing live markers that you correctly identify. Once you have a success, file that experience away so the next time you see that same marker on someone

FOOT READING

else you know what exactly what it means. There is a formula to follow for giving a good interpretation though.

First, ask the client to describe in detail what they are feeling in their feet. Normally, my clients come in with a particular issue that they just cannot get rid of. So, for the first few minutes of the session, before any visual assessment of the feet takes place, I listen. I am specifically listening for their adjectives and key words at this point. Sometimes they ramble and that's totally ok, but every couple sentences they will drop some hot word that clues me in to what I might find in the feet. Once I have an overview of their story, what they are feeling, why they came in and a handful of adjectives to use during our conversation, I then ask my questions.

The second and more specific thing I want to know is about the timeline. The timeline is so key to associating the symptom with a stressor and shedding light on the seemingly random pieces of this story to reveal that everything is in fact connected. I am searching for a start date and any details from then until now that are relevant. Again, the client may veer off track here and begin to babble, but your job is to funnel the conversation by re-asking about what you need to know. Do not underestimate the babble though because their venting builds rapport. Just make sure you finally arrive at the goal of getting your timeline straightened out.

Last, we will proceed to our visual assessment of the feet. Here you want to identify the zones where a marker has appeared. This is why memorizing the meanings of each Horizontal Zone and Vertical Zone of Influence is so important. The meaning of the Horizontal Zone will come first followed by the Vertical Zone. Such as a marker in HZ2 and VZ3; how your chest/shoulder area and your feelings/emotions are being influenced by your upper digestive system and your career. See how I did that? I took both the physical and mental/emotional meaning for the Horizontal Zone where the marker is located and said it was being influenced by the Vertical Zone's physical and mental/emotional meaning – it's that simple.

Bringing the entire story of key words, the timeline and the assessment of the actual marker creates the story. At the end of this section I have some trial cases for you to work with; simple recounts of actual clients for you to start practicing your analytical skills. Remember, this book is meant to be a guide and there is no substitute for a live Foot Reading experience. So, make it your mission to put the following framework into action as you put the vocabulary to use in actual conversations. Good luck!

Using the Right Adjectives and Key Words

Words are powerful. The right words can create a harmonious resonance that delivers deeper meaning into the tone of our consultations. The wrong words can leave a client feeling that you've missed the mark or that your interpretations of the markers present don't add benefit to their recovery process. Finding the right words takes time and practice, but by sticking to the meanings of the zones and drawing from the two methods below you will have a safe framework to practice with built-in accuracy.

Call it like you See it

At the beginning of my Foot Reading endeavors, I would be at a loss for words. Not having developed my elemental vocabulary yet or refined my understanding of the zones, I would fumble for an explanation for what I was seeing. When I was up against a wall, I would simply use the words that came to mind when I bluntly described the marker I was looking at. *Call it like you see it* is now the advice I give to my students all of the time. I am constantly amazed with how successful a simple technique like this really is.

When you see a toe that isn't in alignment, would you describe it as leaning or crooked? Leaning is a word that gives a feeling of slightly bending or of sharing weight, while crooked is synonymous with distorted, jagged and is a more intense word with a more sinister connotation. Does the foot have the appearance of being happy? Sounds weird, but sometimes I see feet that just looks a certain way and the first word that pops into my head based on that initial impression is often quite accurate.

Interesting observations can be made as you use your natural vocabulary to assess how markers look. When this practice is implemented with a healthy amount of compassion for the client and a good deal of self-trust, there is a profound alignment within your off the cuff interpretations. Yes, make sure to stick to the basics of zone theory and elemental language, but incorporating the initial reaction to the feet or marker in front of you can yield surprising results. These words are spontaneous and strong and will get stuck in your head for the whole reading so better to write them down and at least mention them in passing.

This skill harnesses your subconscious data bank of patterns that you have been picking up on your entire lifetime. Eventually, your mental rolodex will merge with the zones and elemental language, creating an ability to shoot from the hip and accurately assess feet on sight. Start by noticing those first one or two key words that jump to mind when looking at a pair of feet for the first time. How would you describe them overall, as tired, energetic, meek, profound, gracious, or well balanced? This is your first clue and can be the gateway for deeper themes to reveal themselves.

Using the Client's Chosen Words

The choice words someone uses reveals much about their character; even more so in the context of a Foot Reading. When a client uses pointed words to describe their current state I will write down or mentally file away exactly what word(s) they used for later mention during the session. The amount of information conveyed by someone's word choice when describing their foot issues, or their feet in general, has great significance in Foot Reading. Adjectives can be thought of as connectors within themselves as clients will often use the same words to describe their physical/mental/emotional state as they describe their particular foot dis-ease.

Does the condition of their feet bother them, irritate them, frustrate them, enrage them, piss them off or is it just there? Did it come on suddenly, gradually, in spurts, overnight or has it always been in the background? Does it make them self-conscious, ashamed, concerned, worried, perplexed, or is it just something they live with? Word choice, word choice, word choice. Beginning the dialogue by asking them why they are bringing their feet to you and to describe in detail what they are concerned about, even if they are just talking generally about their feet, you have got some good information there to use later.

Backing up into elemental language, pay attention to any key words clients use that may give you clues based on what you already know about symptomology. Check out the words below to see how everyday adjectives clients use can describe an elemental presence:

Earth
They feel stiff, hard as a rock, like I'm walking on a pebble, there is a heaviness, immoveable, rough, caveman/cavewoman feet, boney, bigger than they should be (*width*) misshapen, grounded, stuck in the mud, stubborn

Air
I feel ungrounded, can't get my footing, they fly out from under me, needing to be free (*feeling constrained*), always dry, pale, delicate, circulation, light, smaller than they should be (*narrow*), I'm super flexible, so thin, frail, inflated, restless

Fire
Hot, stinging, burning, stabbing, painful, cramping, red, flushed, irritating, inflamed, angry, dynamic, dramatic, bigger than they should be (*length*), curvaceous, muscular, engaged, powerful

Water
Cold, wet, clammy, round, veiny, swollen, puffy, like I'm walking in water, like I'm wearing wet shoes, gentle, sweaty, smelly, smaller than they should be (*short*), tiny feet, deep in there, sensitive

FOOT READING

Developing the Timeline

A marker without context is two-dimensional. Yes, it is located within the intersection of certain Horizontal and Vertical Zones. Yes, there are defining elements present to let you know what type of activity is happening within those zones. Even the foot or feet where the marker is located is significant in terms of right side/left side and past/present. But, there is a dramatic increase in palpable significance when you begin to delve into the actual timeframe when a marker began to present itself and how long it has been present. The trick is to find this timeline and then associate it with a matching internal and external stressor to develop greater meaning and understanding for the owner of the marker.

There is a step-by-step checklist that I go by to determine the extent of the timeline, along with what happened in between the marker presenting and the client seeing me for a session. The conversation begins with the originating time of the marker surfacing. Determining the exact timeframe is very important; not so specific as the day and hour, but making sure to have a clear starting point in mind. Identifying the starting point of the marker is then followed up with a broad question about the consistency of symptoms. Has there been a consistent presence, or has the intensity of the marker increased or decreased over that time?

The conversation often goes something like this:

Me: "When did that pain in the ball of the foot start?"

Client: "Around three months ago."

Me: "Was it consistent in its pain level or did it get worse/better at any time?"

Client: "Well, it was getting better, then it got worse. Then I went to the Podiatrist and they shot it with some cortisone and that worked for a few days, but it's been hurting on and off still and no one can figure out why."

Me: "Interesting. So, what was happening in your life three months ago? Specifically, in relation to your emotions and your chest/shoulder area?"

Client: *After thinking, becomes visibly shocked* "Well, that was when I started a new project at work that I had been asking to take on for a really long time, but it quickly overwhelmed me."

Me: "And when the pain subsided from the ball of the foot, around that time what was happening with the project?"

Client: "Oh, my boss assigned two additional people to help with the project, but we eventually started to disagree about how to execute the tasks needed to get it done. We have good days and bad days."

Me: "Just like with your foot?"

Client: *Hesitant* "...Yeah...."

Me: "And your shoulder?"

Client: "Oh, my massage therapist is taking care of that. It started to get stiff and kind of painful, but I get it worked on every other week which keeps it in check."

Me: "Did the shoulder start about three months ago?"

Client: "Ye-How did you know?"

Me: "Your foot."

Timing is exact within the body. The pervading theory that the internal environment of the body is truly interconnected on a moment to moment basis is the bedrock for this work. Making sure to identify this timeline clearly helps build the bridge between the client and their body; helping them understand this exact link is the key to unwinding the symptom through lifestyle adjustments. When the timeline of symptomology has been discovered and elaborated on, we then move the conversation to the wording used to describe the marker present.

The Visual Assessment

Last, and only after our contextual clues have been collected, we need to visually assess the feet. Another reason why Reflexology as a hands-on modality is so helpful to this process is that during an hour session you as the practitioner get to see, feel and take your time discovering the markers present within the foot. Texture can reveal a more refined nuance dynamics of assessment rather than relying on visual observation alone, but there is an importance to the eye-catching art of visual assessment. When I see a foot for the first time, there is an order I wish to proceed in to make sure that I am able to access a complete picture of all aspects present.

Step One: Placement

At the start, I will have my client first take off their shoes and socks. Clients normally will have cleaned their feet beforehand or gotten a pedicure, but a bathroom nearby is handy if clients need to tidy up their feet pre-assessment. Then, they will lie face up (*as if they were sleeping on their back*) on a massage table. This allows me to assess both the top and bottom surfaces of the feet at once without the client needing to hold up their feet. I will only have them here for a few minutes, enough time for me to jot down my finding. After, we will proceed to a more comfortable sitting position that allows for face to face dialogue.

Step Two: Notice the Big Things

Next, having the client's feet where I want them I will then take a wide-angle view of the larger picture; accurately surveying of the tops and bottoms of the feet. I ask myself questions like: *What strikes me first? What seems out of place? What catches my eye?* After observing both surfaces thoroughly and seeing what there is to see, I will take a clipboard with a piece of paper and pen and writing the three more important markers I see. These are my 'top three' and will be the major talking points for the consultation.

The importance of finding two or three very striking markers serves a few functions. First, these three markers are the most prominent markers meaning that they are issues that the body has vocalized the strongest or spent the most energy to create i.e. a gnarly bunion, large patches of odd skin and/or severe pain. Second, the three big markers are guideposts to keep the coaching dialogue focused on the most pertinent issues and prevent our conversation from straying into smaller topics that aren't as important to address. Often, these smaller markers are side-effects of the larger ones anyways.

You will note that I mentioned pain in the foot as a marker, but you cannot necessarily see pain in the body. Here you will need to rely on the client's testimony paired with what you see in the physical reflexes areas. However, if pain exists but you cannot see signs of it on the outside, that is also significant.

Step Three: The Smaller Things and General Constitutional Themes

Once I've categorized my star players, I being to pick out the lesser markers, nitpicky things and overarching themes within the constitution. Lesser markers are smaller things that you have to look harder to find; the markers that you don't see right away and are therefore not as significant, but are relevant nonetheless. Constitutional themes are also very helpful to identify during a Foot Reading consultation. Sometimes, the fact that someone has a very dominant element in their constitution becomes one of my top three markers because of how present the characteristics of those elemental themes are. Other times, I will only write down that there are slight tilts in balance towards one of the four elements depending on what I see. Now is the time to quickly note the subtler dynamics within the feet.

Step Four: Setting Up to Consult

After I have gathered my information, my client and I proceed to sit down in a comfortable and private area to discuss my findings. Normally, I take a few minutes, but for your first couple of readings on friends and family I would suggest taking more time to make sure you do not miss anything important. The goal is to thoroughly examine the feet, then take that information and translate it into a conversation. Make sure you feel comfortable with the amount of information you have gleaned before proceeding. You can always take another peek if needed, but I prefer to do the assessment quickly so there can be ample time to share and understand.

A Note for Remote Consultations

Again, when I began to do Foot Reading consultations I was asked to do them remotely. There are some problems with this for the beginner who is struggling with the basics. The first issue is that when someone shows you their feet through an online conferencing platform there may be technical or environmental issues such as bad lighting, poor equipment or *(and this has happened to me many times)* the person may not be as good operating the camera on their device. All of the above scenarios and more can interfere with the visual quality of a remote consultation.

For this reason, I recommend you to work with live feet until you feel comfortable conducting a full hour Foot Reading session based on the information you find. Only when you feel confident should an online version be pursued as you will have worked out the kinks. The virtue of patience should also be cultivated for remote video calls because the person is often in their own space which may be interrupted, distracting the process. All of these are simply points to consider before venturing into a less clear medium rather than a live set of feet in front of you.

At this point in the consultation, I have greeted the client, collected valuable information in regards to why they are here, surveyed their feet and we have made ourselves comfortable to begin our discussion of the findings. Notably, the first words out of my client's mouths are: What did you see? Before I even answer their question, there are some tactics I employ to make sure that my words are simple to understand, truthful and pleasing to hear.

Ethical Considerations

Do No Harm

The medical oath I feel directly applies to Foot Reading. Coaching and consulting of any kind should be first and foremost a service with the highest good of the client at the forefront. Because of the environment of this work, you are tapping into dynamics of confidentiality, vulnerability and medically sensitive information. This level of interaction does require seriousness. The goal is always to help and any intention contra to that should be fully discarded before heading into a Foot Reading session.

Now, on the flip side of this seriousness there is the word *consultation*. Practitioners of Foot Reading should not be giving medical advice, should not be prescribing medicine and should not be treating anyone for a specific condition. We are consultants using Reflexology theory to provide a different perspective. It just so happens that people will tell you their life story and sometime confer deep trust. This is because we are willing to listen. However, referring to the appropriate licensed medical professional should be quickly given priority if the consultation uncovers a client's serious concerns.

Take your work seriously, but first and foremost *Do No Harm*.

Keep your Language Simple

I can speak in fancy words and I have a passion for intricate language (*as you may have noticed throughout this book*). I advise you now to keep your language simple and easy to digest for the client you are engaging with. If they don't know what you are trying to say, then your assessment is moot because the message wasn't received. A client must fully understand what you are saying. Sometimes that requires creative analogy, comparisons and storytelling to convey what you have found.

This is one of the main reasons why the meaning of the zones has been boiled down to a few key words. For those of you who understand the chakra system, you will notice some similarities in how the zones are gridded. Other theories and realms of assessment have complicated words, terms, cultural context and meanings that are very difficult for an outsider to understand. The basic elemental language I taught you will work in your favor to this end. Simplify concepts into their elementary state and make sure that you are understood before closing the session.

Say what you See

Part of my journey was misinterpretation and withholding of information that I was uncomfortable vocalizing at the time. There is a fine line to tread here because I do not want to put you in an uncomfortable situation, but I must remind you to say what you see in its entirety if you feel it is within your ability to do so. Too many clients would return to me with stories of struggle that I had clearly seen in their feet, but did not wish to vocalize because I felt that it 'wasn't my place'.

I agree that there is a time and place for everything and that sometimes you should not vocalize when it would be inappropriate. Part of my dysfunction was lacking the information I have now refined over time into this book, but there was also a lack of confidence as well. Believe me, Foot Reading is accurate. Your interpretation may not be spot on or may be a little muddled at times, but I must encourage that saying something despite lingering insecurities is needed.

Temper your Words

Piggybacking off the above statements is the cultivated ability to temper one's words. This includes the ethical breech of diagnosing through the feet, which we *Do Not* do. Word choice is part of the craft and I just advised you to listen intently to the words of your client for information that will help you in your assessment. Before you use a word that may be startling, inflammatory, sharp or emotionally charged, temper your wording. Make sure your client would receive your choice words with the correct intention before using them.

On the flip side of this argument is vague language that needs to be sharpened. Again, the long-time theme of refining your Foot Reading craft bears mention here. Let me warn you that use of ambiguous language or waffling your words will leave the client asking for clarity. Use the practice examples at the end of this chapter to refine your skills and create your own practice scenarios so that you are able to make your word choices more profoundly accurate.

What to Charge

My hands-on Reflexology sessions and my Foot Reading consultations are the same price because it is the same time and energy I am giving to that individual. I charge seventy-five dollars an hour as of this book's publication for an hour session. There are several things wrong with me telling you this, but here are the top three: 1) You are not me and I am not you 2) You do not live where I live demographic-wise 3) Your needs may be different. What you charge should be based off a personal value of your own worth, what the people in your area will be able to pay for your services and what your individual needs are as a person.

To give further clarity, I live and work in South Tampa, Florida. I grew up here and I have a long-standing reputation in the community after being a Reflexologist here for over eight years. I can't go to the grocery store without seeing a client of mine; we are still a smaller city. The income range varies, but there is a wealthier and more business-savvy community here that can support paying seventy-five dollars an hour for my time. Now, I know Foot Readers in New York who charge more and Foot Readers in my area that are providing hour sessions for sixty dollars. I would encourage you to see what local bodyworkers are charging in your area and make sure that, whatever you charge, you are comfortable with that number.

Repeat Clients

Taking a coaching approach to this work requires a focus on results and education. After you have correctly identified the markers present in relationship to the person's state, then the next affair is helping the client identify what would help them bring their current situation back into balance. In most cases there is a good month or two in between my Foot Reading sessions because the client now knows what is happening and how to prevent it. The ball is in their court.

The repeat clients that see me are looking for continued guidance because something isn't sinking in. Either their body continues to manifest the symptom and we need to re-evaluate the meaning or the person isn't doing what they decided to do and we need to re-evaluate that plan. In both cases a follow-up is needed. The problem becomes when no action is taken and the results aren't present. Make sure that your sessions stay focused on the goal and feel free to refer clients who are not receiving the work to another practitioner who would serve them better – there is no shame in this.

Methods of Balancing the Elements

Speaking with clients about what their markers mean based on Reflexology theory is one thing. Educating the client on how they can potentially rearrange their life to bring relief from the elemental imbalances that are plaguing them is another story all together. Once a marker has been identified and the source of stress understood, the next step is to work in a coaching capacity with the client to help them figure out for themselves what would be the most efficient changes to start implementing. The easiest way to do this is by applying the same elemental language and adjectives used to describe the marker to understand what needs to happen to release it.

During the *Elements of a Symptom* section I peppered in some ideas and stories about how I've coached clients with various markers. Let's look at some more focused examples:

Balancing Earth

Earth is the element of *Density*, *Width* and *Growth*. As an element, Earth hoards resources and accumulates energy, which it then packs to create the above qualities. The opposing element of Air has the traits that counterbalance the rigidity of Earth. Instead of hoarding, there needs to be a releasing. Instead of defensiveness, there needs to be a sense of whimsy. Instead of the joints locking into place, there needs to be openness and freedom. Because of all these reasons we are seeking to liberate, inspire and loosen the fixed nature of Earth symptomology.

Modalities like yoga and Thai Massage are very helpful for the stretching and opening effects needed to circulate excess Earth from the tissues. Internally, shaking up the status quo through spontaneous activities can be a great way to get out of old ruts. Trying new things, customizing to the marker present, that help to address specific mental/emotional rough spots can greatly benefit the person suffering from *Infection of Earth* markers. The goal is circulation that helps disperse the hardened energy of the marker at hand.

Balancing Air

As Earth's opposite, Air's qualities mirror Earth perfectly from the other side of the spectrum. *Light, Thin and Circulatory* are the three words to best describe this element and Earth is perfectly poised to help regulate those qualities so they don't get out of hand – as Air often does. The lack of substance helps Air to be free and move from place to place without hesitation, but the tradeoff for lightness is deficiency. This lacking produces a thin frame and more fragile constitution which requires constant nourishment and bolstering from Earth in the form of food calories.

Air markers such as dryness, lines and splits in the tissues of the feet can all be nourished back to health through proper injection of nutrients. Hearty stews are an excellent addition to lifestyle should an Infection of Air be present; also the production of a stricter and more defined (*Earth*) schedule that allows the body to distribute resources evenly. In this schedule, lifting weights at the gym would be an excellent activity because it allows the density of Earth to strengthen the flightier constitution without expending massive amounts of energy like running would or risk stretching an already hypermobile body like yoga or massage would.

Balancing Fire

The way to balance Fire is not to smother it, but to feed it appropriately and protect it from excess. For this reason, Water is not always the most appropriate element to balance Fire. I find that Earth balances Fire far better as it both fuels through nutrients, yet controls through boundaries. Fire infections are often due to deep stores of emotions (*Water*) that have been pressurized and over time, more like oil under the Earth's surface, which has been exposed due to over circulation (*Air*) and provides the perfect fuel for the smallest spark of competition and muscular flexion to become a roaring blaze within the body.

For that reason, guiding the passions and explosions of Fire require the return to things as they were in the immediate moment. Once the Fire has been transformed into the steady hearth it is meant to be, then the deeper issues of suppressed emotion can be addressed. Suggesting the client formalize their routines and engage in activities that are productive, but to some degree monotonous, will help the excess Fire burn away and help set a positive framework should this ignition happen again. Avoid the urge to fight Fire with Water; the goal is not to extinguish, leaving an empty scorched shell, but to support and mend through structured care.

Balancing Water

Similar to how Water should not balance Fire in the body, so too should Water not balance Fire – all you do is create steam which adds to pressure. Instead, I find that Air balances Water nicely. Water's tendencies in the body are to stagnate and coagulate. When Water becomes an issue, it is directly related to a lack of circulation which is the domain of Air. Once circulation is established, then the appropriate controls (*Earth*) and passions (*Fire*) can return, but first the swamp must be drained through movement. The elemental balance can be easily restored in the short term through movement of any kind, manual or exercise-related, so the enemy of isolated stillness can be overcome.

The discharge of anxious and cold feelings that excess Water produces is first priority. Fire as Water's opposite cannot exist in such a damp environment. Once the fluid and emotions are taken care of, then further elemental balancing can come into play. As someone who was a very Watery constitution, I can personally attest to how important any kind of physical activity is when my internal and physical environment becomes waterlogged. You can literally feel as if you are drowning in yourself, but the first course of action should always be to move, move, and move so you can see what is lurking in the depths that caused the flood to begin in the first place.

Use your Tool Kit

Everyone has a different set of skills and experiences. Use what you have! I am speaking about my own observations when explaining how to balance the elemental symptoms, but you may have different ideas. You may be good with essential oils, herbal medicine, Western medicine, personal training, bone adjustment, massage, etc. All of those methods have many levels of practice and I am not equipped to speak about those nuances here, but I would encourage you to find the method that resonates with you and see its effects on friends, family and clients who are suffering with out of control elements.

I'm sure that I've covered the elements thoroughly enough to give

FOOT READING

you an idea of what I'm talking about during assessment, but the suggestions you give should be your own. The confidence to guide someone else will be based on your own experiences and the most powerful guidance comes from developing those experiences over time. If you are particularly gifted with food preparation and manipulating the elements of the body through diet by all means USE THAT! The purpose of this book is to give you the framework to start practicing the principles within. Make sure your voice is your own.

Sample Client Scenarios

These examples are from real clients of mine that helped me define my own boundaries during pressing ethical situations where I questioned myself. That self-inquiry is where the magic happens to make you a better Foot Reader. How would you coach someone who doesn't want to be coached? How can you change your words to better suit a client's unique personality? Those questions and so much more can come up during your consultations, so it is best to prepare for them now with these mock examples to build your critical thinking skills.

Feel free to think up your own examples of how a Foot Reading may take an unexpected turn. Running through the following scenarios in your head and seeing how you would deal with them is an excellent way to practice handling the different dynamics of clients coming in for your assessment skills.

Session Scenario One

Christopher comes to you for advice on chronic callousing on his feet paired with complaints of overall achiness throughout his body. The client's foot is blockish in shape and is presenting a series of callouses all across Horizontal Zone Two on both feet. The ankles are evenly stiff and there is a resonating thickness throughout the foot. What can you tell about Christopher's condition based on this information and how would you convey it to him in a way that matches his constitution?

Session Scenario Two

Julie is a high powered executive woman who has a natural gas pedal foot and a red tint to her skin tone. She came in complaining of fatigue and joint discomfort, specifically in the lower back and shoulders. During the session you notice that Horizontal Zone Three is congested and hot while all the other zones seem slightly cold and loose. She wants actionable steps to implement change in her life, but relays that she could barely make time for the consultation today and isn't sure she can accommodate dramatic lifestyle changes. How would you work with Julie's limited timeframe?

Session Scenario Three

Bob is a handyman with a right foot that constantly cramps. He is coming to you for a combination of Foot Reflexology and a Foot Reading Consultation to aid this issue. You notice during the session that the right foot has raised and hardened the thick plantar tendon in Vertical Zones Two & Three within Horizontal Zone Three. Bob's left foot is actually more puffy and hot than the right foot overall. How would you explain to Bob what his feet are trying to say?

Session Scenario Four

Patricia is an elderly lady just looking to relax with Reflexology session. During the session you notice multiple markers such as clawed toes, arthritic ankles, thickened nails and deep lining Horizontal Zone Two. She thoroughly enjoyed the session and slept through most of it. Would you engage in a deeper dialogue with Patricia?

Session Scenario Five

Ross is an avid golfer who is coming in with a chronic right hip condition. He reports pain and stiffness that is hindering his game to the point that he can barely play. He has spent great amounts of time and money to figure out what it wrong with his body, to no avail. During the session you find swelling in the low back reflexes at Horizontal Zone Four & Vertical Zone One. However, he denies any low back issues and feels your feedback is not helpful. How should this situation be handled?

Session Scenario Six

Christina is a new client referral from a previous client that claims you pinpointed the cause of her acid reflux symptoms in one assessment. Christina has chronic migraines and verbally states to you that she wants you to take them away for her. During the assessment you find a combination of weakness in the dorsal ankles, slight swelling around the medial malleoli and she also has a slight skin condition in Horizontal Zone Four & Vertical Zone One. There are no issues presenting within the toes. What boundaries would need to be drawn before discussing the surprising markers you see?

Session Scenario Seven

Barry was sent to you by a friend of yours who insisted that he get his feet read by you. Barry is skeptical and borderline nervous, but shows up anyways with arms crossed and not saying much. He warms up slightly with an initial dialogue, but does not reveal any details to you about why he is really there. During the assessment you find shedding skin on the right big toe pad, callousing on the right ball of the foot only and shedding on the left heel. Taking into consideration Barry's reservation, how would you change your wording or temperament to put him at ease while conveying the markers present?

Documenting your Foot Reading Consultations

I am not a fan of documentation personally. I've never liked that process and it has been difficult living in the state of Florida where the Western medical system has reached a state of internal dysfunction, which eventually spirals into incompetence. Reflexology and Foot

Reading are a hands-on and discussion approach, respectively. You may want to document your sessions to chart your progress as an assessment specialist or simply to CYA if your area is like mine in regards to regulations. Either way, I encourage you to test out the forms I have listed in this section and as with all material in the book I hope you find it valuable.

These forms are in a SOAP Note format. ***SOAP*** is an acronym for the four steps in documenting the experience you and your client have together.

- ***S*** stands for ***Subjective***; helping you to listen intently to what each client reports to you and using their words to fuel your sessions.
- ***O*** stands for ***Objective***; the markers and details you notice during the exchange.
- ***A*** stands for ***Assessment***; which we have already discussed in depth, here we de-code what markers we find in a written format.
- ***P*** stands for ***Plan***; after the discussion of each marker and its meaning has transpired, what is the plan to correcting the imbalance that the feet are trying to vocalize?

After the blank form I've included for visual reference in this chapter, I've also included three different example forms with fictitious data to help you understand exactly how to document your Foot Reading consultations. The thing that is missing from our Foot Reading SOAP Note is my favorite part of the Foot Reading documentation process: pictures of the markers. Not every marker is photographable, such as pain that has no visible trace, but the ones that are can serve many purposes. Proof is the most obvious, proof that Foot Reading, the markers and zones can in fact map the physical/mental/emotional states of a person.

In addition to basic proof to yourself and others as a way to validate your Foot Reading studies, pictures attached to a Foot Reading SOAP Note can be excellent for future classes you give, papers you publish,

FOOT READING

educating other clients and/or jogging your memory when you know you've seen the marker before, but are struggling with its meaning. Cross-referencing previous sessions with current ones is an excellent way to supercharge your skills. Finally, noting will help you reinforce the fundamentals and can act as a very real focal point to assist you during your first consultations. You will notice that I only include the Top Three markers I see on each documentation form – that is by design to keep you focused on what matters.

Without further ado, may I present the Foot Reading SOAP Note form:

Foot Reading SOAP Note Form

Client:_____

Date:_____

Subjective

Reason for Consultation:

Timeline:

Feedback (*Post-Discussion*):

Observations

Marker 1:

Marker 2:

Marker 3:

Assessment

Marker 1:

Physical:

Mental/Emotional:

Marker 2:

Physical:

Mental/Emotional:

Marker 3:

Physical:

Mental/Emotional:

*P*lan

Methods of Balancing:

Foot Reading SOAP Note Form
EXAMPLE 1

Client: Mary Sue

Date: 7/1/2017

*S*ubjective

Reason for Consultation: Client has long-time foot problems that seem to have gotten worse recently and she is interested to find out why.

Symptomology: Client is reporting arthritis in the second and third toes on the right foot as the major source of her discomfort. The feelings are achy, stiff and slightly swollen. There is also arch tightness occasionally, but the toes are the major pain point.

Timeline: The toes started to hurt when she was in her late teens, but have been off and on since then.

Feedback (*Post-Discussion*): Client reported that she is in a profession that she never wanted to get into, but it pays the bills. She often wonders whether pursuing her dream job would have led to less stress and greater fulfillment. She agreed to incorporate the discussed scheduling of meals and self-care. She will report after a week to relay any change.

Observations

Marker 1: 2nd and 3rd right toes are reported to be achy, stiff and slightly swollen.

Marker 2: A patch of dryness is present on the left foot across the plantar surface of Horizontal Zone Three.

Marker 3: The heels of both feet are redder in color than the rest of the feet, slightly wider and more pronounced.

Assessment

Marker 1:

Physical: Right side chest/lung reflex area and upper digestive area are influencing the neck to become achy, stiff and slightly swollen.

Mental/Emotional: Past thoughts about feelings and career/actions are continuing to emotionally ache (achy and swollen) internally due to a stubbornness (stiff) perspective.

Marker 2:

Physical: Exhaustion in the stomach reflex from sporadic dietary patterns.

Mental/Emotional: Current career stress that is causing a lack of boundaries (Air) and an unpredictable schedule.

Marker 3:

Physical: The sciatic and lower body reflexes are slightly inflamed and agitated.

Mental/Emotional: There is a constant theme of needing to go-go-go.

Plan

Methods of Balancing: Working from the ground up, the client should consider slowing down and planning her schedule as to not miss meals and incorporate time for structured rest. The past thoughts should respond to the planned decompression by releasing the toe symptoms which are caused by past career decisions bubbling to the surface due to the current level of overload.

Foot Reading SOAP Note Form
EXAMPLE 2

Client: John Personable

Date: 7/1/2017

Subjective

Reason for Consultation: Client is reporting sever pain and spasm in the arch (*Horizontal Zone Four & Vertical Zone One*) of this left foot. It wakes him up during the night and seems to be worse in the evenings.

Timeline: The arch started cramping two months ago (*beginning of May*) and has been consistent. He went to get a shot from his Podiatrist for the pain, but it lasted maybe two days and then the cramping returned. The darkened nail found during observation happened about a month ago, it has changed little from the initial injury.

Feedback (*Post-Discussion*): Client reported that his daughter announced her engagement two months ago to get married for the second time and there is great debate over the details of the marriage. Family is extremely important to him and he is having difficulty accepting the non-traditional way that this family situation is being carried out. His lower back has also been seizing up on the left side. Client said he doesn't feel comfortable with yoga, but he will investigate methods of spinal stretching and will get back to writing as his preferred way to calm his mind.

FOOT READING

Observations

Marker 1: Left medial arch at Horizontal Zone Four & Vertical Zone One is painful and with spasm. The area is visibly puffy, hot and has a reddish tint to the skin as well.

Marker 2: Client has a darkened big toe nail on the left foot.

Marker 3: The right medial arch is puffy with raised vasculature. The feet have raised vasculature throughout, but it is most prominent on the arches.

Assessment

Marker 1:

Physical: Left lower back reflex pain and spasm.

Mental/Emotional: Current thoughts influencing family/relationships to become inflamed about two months ago.

Marker 2:

Physical: Left side head/sinus congestion.

Mental/Emotional: Current darkened thoughts that surfaced about a month ago.

Marker 3:

Physical: A constitutional element of stagnant fluid within the spinal reflex that needs to be circulated regularly.

Mental/Emotional: Client's thoughts are highly sensitive and needs more physical/internal self-care in this area of life.

Plan

Methods of Balancing: The current family stress cannot be avoided, but the stress itself needs to be channeled properly. Client's body has always stagnated in the spinal reflexes. Seeing a Chiropractor and developing a yoga practice for spinal health would be an ideal combination to both decompress physically and help release internal tensions.

Foot Reading SOAP Note Form
EXAMPLE 3

Client: <u>Sheila Sun</u>

Date:<u> 7/1/2017</u>

Subjective

<u>Reason for Consultation:</u> Client has developed a skin condition on her feet that has her worried.

<u>Symptomology:</u> Client is reporting itchy and irritated patches of skin that have appeared in the creases between the toes into the top of the right foot and a recent diagnosis of a Morton's Neuroma on the left foot.

<u>Timeline:</u> The skin condition has been off and on for six months now and the Morton's Neuroma has only developed over the past two weeks, although she has had the issue before on the same foot six years ago.

<u>Feedback (*Post-Discussion*):</u> Client reported that she is currently emotionally struggling to define herself. The anniversary of her own mother's passing was last month (*the six-year anniversary*) and it brought the need to reflect on her roles as a daughter, a mother and a caregiver for her father.

She reports all of this hitting her at the beginning of the year when her child left for college and she is now an empty-nester; the tension has been slowly building since she now has the time to reminisce.

Observations

<u>Marker 1</u>: Right foot presents red, itchy and irritated on the dorsal surface between the toes at the base of Horizontal Zone One and into the top of Horizontal Zone Two – straddling the Shoulder Line Guideline.

Marker 2: Morton's Neuroma pain on the left ball of the foot in Horizontal & Vertical Zone Two with visible puffiness.

Marker 3: There is an inward plantar wart on the right ball of the foot in Horizontal & Vertical Zone Two. Client did not feel it was important to mention.

Assessment

Marker 1:

Physical: Irritated and inflamed tissue in the upper back and lower neck on the right side.

Mental/Emotional: Past irritating thoughts about feelings that started six months ago.

Marker 2:

Physical: Impingement in the left chest/shoulder complex, same physical issue that happened six years ago.

Mental/Emotional: Current emotional pain that is being kept under the surface, which is most likely a re-surfacing of the same emotional pain experienced six years ago.

Marker 3:

Physical: Deep weakness (*Air*) and stagnation (*Water*) in the right shoulder complex.

Mental/Emotional: Previous sorrow and emotional vulnerability regarding past events is being hold onto.

Plan

Methods of Balancing: Since all markers are heavily related to Horizontal Zone Two, the targeted area of self-care should be the chest and shoulder complex on both sides. Gentle physical activity that stimulates breathing and use of the arms should be utilized to help release physical and emotional tension. Working with a counselor or advisor is suggested to establish a firm support system that helps unwind both the surface and underlying emotions connected to past stressors.

Generating a Foot Reading Report

Consultations can be given live in-person or online through various video conferencing platforms. Another useful tool I have created is for a client who would like to know what is happening in their feet, but would prefer to have a written report in addition to, or instead of, a live or online consultation. For this purpose, I began to create Foot Reading Reports where I take photos given to me by clients and document my findings in a written format that I then email to them for a fee – the cost of which I charge forty-five dollars for. The report itself is about one thousand words long, about three pages without fancy formatting, and includes a few helpful additives that I will now explain.

Introduction & Key Points

When typing a report, the first thing I write is a thank you for purchasing the report. This goes a long way in making the client feel like you are as happy to create the report as they are to purchase it. In the introduction I also add a little bit about how the report should be read and the section within. The intention of any intro is to prepare the reader as best as possible to digest the contents of the report and understand how to read the details.

Below the introduction, but before we get into the meat of the report, I like to include some *Key Points*. Once I look at the pictures for a few minutes and I get the general layout of what markers I want to talk about, I'll use the key points section to prime the reader with a little bit of Foot Reading knowledge to give better context for what is about to come. Defining key words and concepts before delving into the markers helps set the stage and makes the recipient more of an educated consumer before proceeding.

Circle the Markers

The bulk of the report itself contains the marker interpretations and meanings present within the pictures that were sent. To emphasize and outline what I am talking about, I will take the picture into a word or paint program and draw colored circles around the markers I will be referencing. This helps to take the visual burden off the client who normally has no idea what we as Foot Readers are looking at unless the markers are really prominent. Just like in a consultation, you want to make sure that you only choose your Top Three markers to focus on; less and the report may seem a little sparse, but more can equally overwhelm.

Picture quality is important here because you do want to show something substantial that the client can see with their own eyes. Sometimes I will ask clients to send better quality pictures or re-take them in better lighting so I can show them a clearer image of what I see. The goal for me is to give a tangible feeling to the client of seeing what I see. Foot Reading when done by report is all about the visuals, so make sure your targets are easy to see for both you and your client.

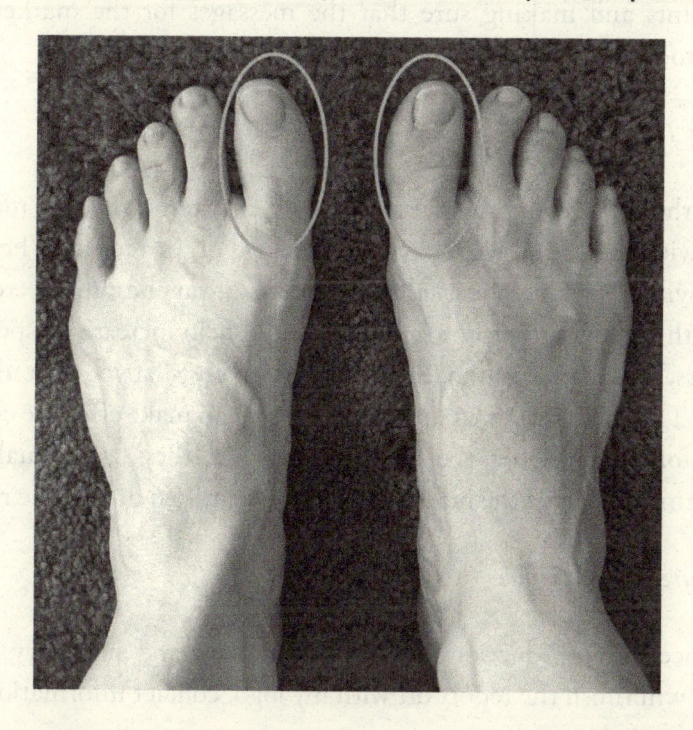

Explain Each Marker's Meaning

Just like in our SOAP Notes, both the physical and mental/emotional meanings are given for each marker. This point needs to be driven home because not including both meanings will jip your clients of information that may move the needle for them. Some clients say they only want to know the physical aspects, others want just the internal meanings, but everyone needs to hear both sides of the story; especially since you want to be as thorough as possible because the report is written and not verbal.

Summary

Towards the end of the report, after all the markers are explained in depth, I will add a paragraph summary to tie everything together. Normally, this includes whittling down the details into a more refined few sentences. This gives your client a focused take-away of everything you have said so far. In the summary you are hammering home the key points and making sure that the messages for the markers are understood.

Closing Tips

At the risk of sounding overly critical, I counterbalance the markers I find with three solid wellness tips at the end of the report. When you are relaying how someone is falling apart it is always best to sweeten the end with some healthy protocols that would help increase the person's wellness, which are customized to them based on what you have already found. This is similar to having an action plan to make effective change going forward; leaving the client feeling like they can actually do something to change the markers you have identified during the report.

Signature & Disclaimer

Once the introduction, key points, markers and summary are in place I will finish the report off with my logo, contact information and a disclaimer at the bottom to avoid being pegged as giving diagnosis, prescription or treatment. This statement reads something like this:

PLEASE NOTE: *This report is not intended to Diagnose, Prescribe and/or Treat any physical, mental and/or emotional medical condition. The report is only meant to assess, coach and educate the recipient on Reflexology theory. If you have a genuine medical concern, it is best to consult a physician to ensure properly licensed care.*

The benefits of generating such a report for a client, when charging or just working with friends and family, are manifold. Professionalism is the first benefit that comes to my mind. When clients hear of my Foot Reading Consultations, I get weird looks. Showing those same clients an example of a neat, thorough and fascinating report changes their opinion of Foot Reading in an instant. Is does take some computer skills and the ability to translate your thoughts into written word, but the efficiency and high quality of such a report really impresses prospective clients.

In addition to wooing over your database, you are documenting your Foot Reading experiences in a fun way that you can catalogue for future use; instruction being top of mind for me. You are providing valuable insight and building your repertoire at the same time! The next time a client comes in with a marker you have already profiled as part of your report, you can simply show them the meaning associated and it affirms for the client that you aren't just pulling the meaning out of thin air. When you have documented proof, including feedback from the client you generated the report for there is a palpable wow-factor that is injected into the conversation.

Section Recap

- Remember to **use your client's words** and elemental language to help in your assessment.
- **A timeline is extremely important** for developing an accurate association for when the physical, mental and emotional stressors took place.
- Conducting a visual assessment occurs in the order of: **Placement, Finding the Big Things, then the Smaller Things, General Constitutional Themes and then preparing to Consult.**
- **Keep ethical standards high** when conducting a Foot Reading Consultation.
- **Use your own toolkit** when seeking to balance the elements, but remember that it is not as simple as balancing through opposites as the body is dynamic.
- Documenting your experiences can occur through **SOAP Notes and generating Foot Reading Reports.**

Exploring the Other Extremities

I couldn't stop at just the feet – the body wouldn't let me. Once I became proficient at reading the feet, I was brought a series of clients who displayed prominent markers on the hands, face and ears as well. This was perplexing to me and I felt a deep asking from the body to explore the zones of Reflexology on other surfaces. Using the map that I've already outlined in this book and using my clients as test subjects, I proceeded to occasionally analyze the markers on the hands, face and ears with astounding results: it all worked. This revelation was both exciting and disturbing on many levels.

The first roadblock I had to encounter was that I was the 'foot guy'. Branching into the other extremities required additional explanation that I still wasn't comfortable with discussing at the time, but the hands, face and ears gave me markers that I just couldn't ignore. I still use feet as my primary source of assessment, hence the focus of this book on the feet, but I do respect that the other extremities do have a voice of their own and I would be remiss if I did not include that voice here. There are also nuances I've learned along the way that may be helpful as you explore mapping the other surfaces I outline.

The major purpose of this section for me is because of the students I've taught. In my classes there are students who seem to be drawn to a particular extremity with a gravitational pull that surpasses the others. I respect this natural inclination and understand that I have found my niche in the feet, but that others may find another extremity more valuable. For this reason, I have added this section of the book to inspire the next generation of Hand Readers, Face Readers and Ear Readers who may find this content the most valuable part of this text.

Just as the feet have called me to uncover their mysteries, you may be beaconed by a different surface. The mapping system I've already outlined in this book will be applied just as it exists on the feet. This gives you an easily transferable knowledge base to begin exploring the other extremities while using the vocabulary and grid that I have hopefully drilled into your head up until this point. The challenge will be gaining your own experience, which I cannot provide in this text. I have worked extensively with the feet, but I only claim to dabble in the other extremities as they are not my life's work. Still, the knowledge is sound and I have validated it; it is just not as much my work as it may be yours.

Before we get into the details of each extremity, let me warn you about the differences in markers that are present on the feet, versus the hands, versus the face, versus the ears. Each extremity can be likened to a witness of a car accident standing on a different corner of the same intersection – they all see a slightly different side of the story. Although they will agree that an issue is taking place in the body, the details each extremity focuses on seems to be slightly different in accordance with the physical and energetic function; more on this as we outline each extremity individually.

Mapping the Hands

So, do you read the future? That is the common question I get asked when I talk about reading the extremities in general, but even more so when referencing the hands. Hand Reflexology is a stand-alone branch of the hands-on and assessment technique; I have students that choose to only practice this side of the work. However, there is no similarity to Palmistry as we only see past stressors still being held in the body and the present activity of a person. Likewise, we do not factor in the major lines of the hands; we do assess the lining present on the hands as an Air marker, but not the significance of a life line, heart line, etc.

The hands have their own flavor that colors their message in alignment with their form, function and location. The hands are mobile and Airy structures that allow us to hold, release, fiddle, sculpt, touch and speak in accordance with our will in the present moment. They are an extension of Horizontal Zone Two by location which means that the hands are extremely influenced by feelings and emotions along with all of the structures in the zone: shoulders, chest, ribs, thoracic spine, lungs, heart, and arms. Although the hands will manifest the same general or acute issues as the other extremities, the hands have a more emotional and upper body flavor to the markers they carry.

For instance, the hands will manifest arthritic fingers in the presence of still thoughts that are emotionally influenced and neck issues that have a heavy shoulder component. If someone's injury or dis-ease has a strong heart center influence, then there may be a more visual marker on the hands than the other three extremities. I have learned that the hands also obtain and release markers quicker than the other extremities because the hands are more circulatory in nature. All of these little nuances have surfaced as I have questioned why the hands seem to be more vocal during certain Foot Reading sessions.

The mapping for the zones, the elemental markers and coaching aspects remain entirely the same. The only major difference is the surface you are looking at as the hands have different (*yet still strikingly similar*) bone structure compared to the feet. Another minor difference is the use of anatomical position terms, but the reflexes stay the same. Let's outline the location of the Guidelines, Horizontal and Vertical Zones, and their respective meanings similar to how we did for the feet at the beginning of this book, but with a little more speed as you know the basics already:

SAM BELYEA

HAND HORIZONTAL & VERTICAL ZONES

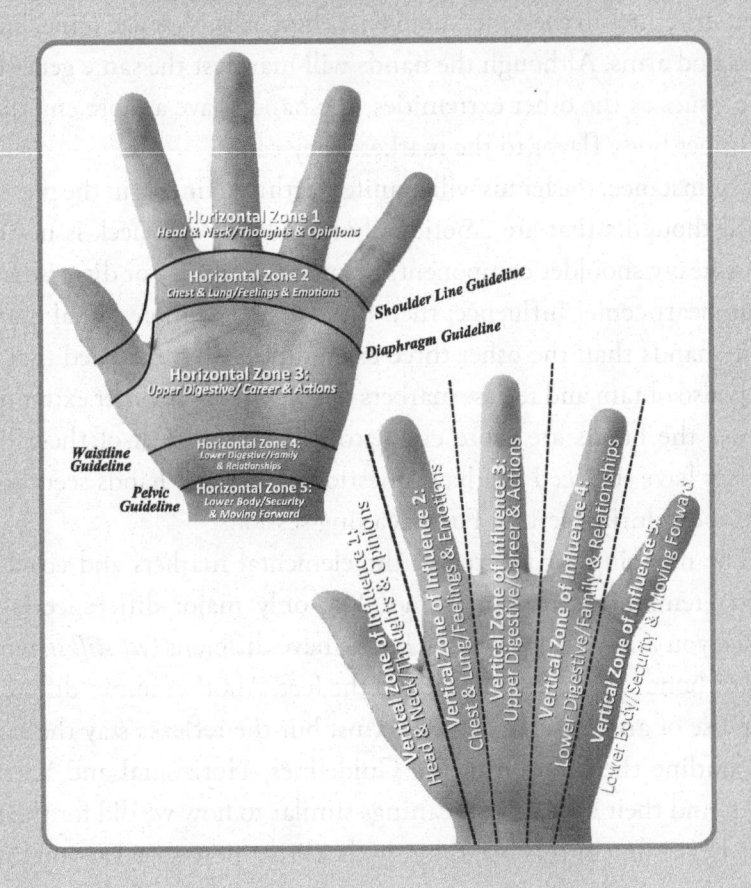

Horizontal Zone 1: Head & Neck/Thoughts & Opinions
Horizontal Zone 2: Chest & Lung/Feelings & Emotions
Shoulder Line Guideline
Diaphragm Guideline
Horizontal Zone 3: Upper Digestive/Career & Actions
Waistline Guideline
Horizontal Zone 4: Lower Digestive/Family & Relationships
Pelvic Guideline
Horizontal Zone 5: Lower Body/Security & Moving Forward

Vertical Zone of Influence 1: Head & Neck/Thoughts & Opinions
Vertical Zone of Influence 2: Chest & Lung/Feelings & Emotions
Vertical Zone of Influence 3: Upper Digestive/Career & Actions
Vertical Zone of Influence 4: Lower Digestive/Family & Relationships
Vertical Zone of Influence 5: Lower Body/Security & Moving Forward

Shoulderline Guideline:

The imaginary line that divides the head and neck structures from the chest, lung and shoulder area. Likewise, dividing the fingers from the knuckles of the hand by drawing a line at the intersection between where the fingers grow out from the hand.

Diaphragm Guideline:

The imaginary line that divides the chest, lung and shoulder area from the structures of the upper digestive system and upper core. Likewise, dividing the knuckles of the hand from the distal (*farther from the body*) palm of the hand by drawing a line below the distal heads of the metacarpals.

Waistline Guideline:

An imaginary line that divides the upper core from the structures of the lower core and pelvic area. Likewise, dividing the proximal (*closer to the body*) palm of the hand from the heel of the hand by drawing a line from the proximal head of the 5th metacarpal across the width of the palm.

Pelvic Guideline:

An imaginary line that divides the lower core and pelvic structures from the lower body. Likewise, dividing the heel of the hand from the wrist by drawing a line in between the two rows of carpal bones.

Horizontal Zone One

<u>Location:</u> The Fingers
<u>Guideline:</u> Shoulderline
<u>Physical Reflexes Present:</u> All structures of the head, neck and face. Including: Brain, Skull, Sinus, Eyes*, Teeth, Jaw, Ears*, Thyroid, Cervical Spine, Muscles/Bones of the Head and Face
<u>Mental/Emotional Meaning:</u> Thoughts and Opinions

To Reinforce: The fingers are equivalent to the toes and represent the exact same structures head and neck. The same conversation can be had about the nails of the fingers representing the soft tissues of the face and the screen of the mind.

Horizontal Zone Two

Location: The Knuckles
Guideline: Shoulderline & Diaphragm
Physical Reflexes Present: Shoulder, Lung, Heart (*more left side*), Ribs, Thymus, Breast, Arm*, Diaphragm (*technically on the Diaphragm Guideline*), Lymph Drainage, Upper Half of Thoracic Spine, Muscles/Bones of the Chest
Mental/Emotional Meaning: Feelings and Emotions

To Reinforce: Here we have to get creative because the hand is structured differently from the foot, plus there is greater space between the thumb and index finger along with a size difference. The guidelines take a fun like swoop in Horizontal Zone Two to create continuity as we jump from the index finger to the thumb, but other than that difference everything is the same. Interesting to note that where the thumb joins the hand it will protrude and swell just like the bunion of the big toe. For this reason, I will call the lower thumb joint the bunion of the hand.

Horizontal Zone Three

Location: The Palmar Surface
Guideline: Diaphragm & Waistline
Physical Reflexes Present: Liver (*right hand*), Gallbladder (*right hand*), Pancreas (*more left hand*), Stomach (*left hand*), Spleen (*left hand*), Adrenal, Upper Half of Kidneys, Solar Plexus (*technically on Diaphragm Guideline*), Lower Half of Thoracic Spine, Muscles/Bones of the Upper Core
Mental/Emotional Meaning: Career and Actions

To Reinforce: The hands have a lot of space in the palmar surface dedicated to Horizontal Zone Three. I do find that the hands are very quick to influence upper digestive distress and I have worked with many hands-on Reflexology clients to alleviate acute digestive distress through the hands. The hands are often the major tool of work which could add to the meaning, but one could also argue that the feet are as well depending on the task at hand. Another factor to consider is that I have noticed many consultation clients with hands that display skin conditions from dietary influences.

From a purely physical perspective, Horizontal Zone Three in the hand runs the length of the metacarpal bones of the hand. The switch in orientation also needs to be observed depending on the direction the hands are facing when being assessed; that threw me for a loop at first. This zone is probably the trickiest to nail down in terms of difference from the feet.

Horizontal Zone Four

<u>Location:</u> Heel of the Hand
<u>Guideline:</u> Waistline & Pelvic
<u>Physical Reflexes Present:</u> Large Intestine (*ascending and half of transverse on right hand; descending, sigmoid and half of transverse on left hand*), Small Intestine, Uterus/Prostate (*lateral*), Fallopian Tubes/Vas Deferens (*dorsal*), Ovaries/Testes (*medial*), Hip Joint (*medial styloid process*) Ureters, Bladder, Lower Half of Kidneys, Inguinal Lymph Drainage, Lumbar Spine, Muscles/Bones of the Lower Core
<u>Mental/Emotional Meaning:</u> Family and Relationships

To Reinforce: Horizontal Zone Four in the feet is shaped very different from Horizontal Zone Four in the hands because of function. In the feet, the ankle complex is spring-loaded to provide transference of momentum. This requires a different positioning of the ankle bones which represent the physical hip reflexes. In the hands, the styloid processes of the wrists are situated more in Horizontal Zone Five. However, I've listed it in this zone because of simplicity and the fact that the hips themselves are in Horizontal Zone Four within the body.

Another directional mapping mishap that I made in the beginning is mistaking the medial and lateral or inside and outside reflexes within the hand; we are using Western anatomical position with palms facing forward. In the feet, the big toe and Vertical Zone One is medial or at the midline of the body, but the thumbs and Vertical Zone One in anatomical position for the hands are splayed laterally. Make sure to check out additional Reflexology mapping resources like the charts I've personally designed for more information and a visual representation.

Horizontal Zone Five

Location: Wrist
Guideline: Pelvic
Physical Reflexes Present: Sciatic Nerve, Sacral Spine, Coccyx, Muscles/Bones of the Legs/Low Body
Mental/Emotional Meaning: Sense of Security and Moving Forward

To Reinforce: The second row of carpals in the hand represent Horizontal Zone Five. Because you can't see them or palpate them easily, it is best to imagine the Pelvic Guideline as half way between the proximal head of the 5th metacarpal and the wrist bone. I find it telling that the hands do not have as much lower body zone substance. Back to what I said about flavors and the function of each extremity; the hands are light, mobile and seem to be focused on what's happing in the upper body.

Vertical Zone One

Location: In Line with the Thumb
Physical Influences: All reflexes found in Horizontal Zone One
Mental/Emotional Influence: Thoughts and Opinions

To Reinforce: The thumb and its muscles are the most common reason why a client comes to see me for Hand Reflexology. Also, during a Foot Reading if hand pain is present it is most commonly found in Vertical Zone One. Dis-ease in this zone represents the postural tug of war with the head and neck versus the rest of the body. Internally, the ancient struggle between the mind and the other more survival-based centers of the body.

Vertical Zone Two

<u>Location:</u> In Line with the Index Finger
<u>Physical Influences:</u> All reflexes found in Horizontal Zone Two
<u>Mental/Emotional Influence:</u> Feelings and Emotions

To Reinforce: When the index finger, or any hand structure in line with it, acquires any elemental marker there is a supercharged essence of Horizontal Zone Two influence. The hands are already flavored by this zone due to their location in the body, so when this Vertical Zone becomes active there is a very strong presence of chest, shoulder, heart, lung, feelings and emotional disturbance afoot (*or rather, ahand*)

Vertical Zone Three

<u>Location:</u> In Line with the Middle Finger
<u>Physical Influences:</u> All reflexes found in Horizontal Zone Three
<u>Mental/Emotional Influence:</u> Career and Actions

To Reinforce: When clients come in with contracture of the hand tendons, I see Vertical Zone Three more than any other zone contracture. This would indicate a collapse of the upper digestive reflexes and a loss of one's sense of purpose. When we flip someone off using our middle finger we are effectively saying *My action, will, and drive is better than yours*. Looking deeper into other forms of energetic assessment we can see similarities between the Solar Plexus chakra as the center for power/anger/joy and the attribution of this Vertical Zone to be the influences of those internal forces.

Vertical Zone Four

<u>Location:</u> In Line with the Ring Finger
<u>Physical Influences:</u> All reflexes found in Horizontal Zone Four
<u>Mental/Emotional Influence:</u> Family and Relationships

To Reinforce: Amazing how our customs have developed to sit a ring indicating marriage within Vertical Zone Four as the influence of family and relationships. In addition, this Vertical Zone represents the influence of all pelvic structures.

Vertical Zone Five

<u>Location:</u> In Line with the Little Finger
<u>Physical Influences:</u> All reflexes found in Horizontal Zone Five
<u>Mental/Emotional Influence:</u> Sense of Security and Moving Forward

To Reinforce: Although small, just like its cousin the fifth digit on the feet, the little finger on the hand represents the influence of the entire lower body. Just like with the balls of the feet having the shoulder reflex in Vertical Zone Five, the hands have the shoulder reflex in Horizontal Zone Two and Vertical Zone Five as well.

Mapping the Face

The face was the catalyst that began my initial decent into the underground of further mapping of the non-foot extremities. It all started when a networking partner of mine showed up to a breakfast meeting with a gigantic blemish on his left upper cheek in what would be Horizontal Zone Three. I knew that the body was telling me something and my curiosity had reached dangerously curious levels. So, I asked inquisitively if his stomach had been bothering him around the time the blemish appeared. He responded with an enthusiastic, *"Oh yeah! It was all coming up last night and the night before. I just couldn't keep my food down."* I responded, all too cheerfully with *"Perfect! And what about the blow-up at work that happened recently?"* That is when he stopped, looked at me with an openly puzzled and slightly scared expression and asked, *"How do you know all of this!?"*

At that moment, I knew I had cracked the code for the universal mapping of the extremities and I haven't stopped proving it since then. The face as an extremity has been one of the most fascinating to study because of its position in the body. In mainstream culture, we don't cover the face. Shoes go over feet, gloves or pockets conceal the hands, and hair or a hat can disguise the ears, but the face is always exposed and forward – making it the most fun extremity to read without people looking at you like you're crazy. When you learn to accurately impose the zones onto the face an entire world opens up that lets you know more about a person, more than they probably want you to know, within the first few seconds of meeting them.

As an extremity, the flavor of the ears and face is heavily reflective of Horizontal Zone One. Also, then the body chooses to manifest a marker on the face itself there is an energetic language of needing to literally *face something* that is being suppressed. For this reason, I often think of the face as a whistleblower extremity. We can effectively hide the other three, but when the body wants your attention is a very real way it will put something on your face to show it. The meaning of markers on the face can then take on the additional interpretation of being *top of mind* to the person you are reading.

From a mapping perspective, we are only concerned with the visible portion of the face from the hairline to the jaw. I do not read the scalp, although I may one day venture into it and I know there are schools of scalp reading out there. For now, I want to work with the surface of the extremity that I can readily see. Unlike the other three extremities, the face only has one surface and the right/left sides are conjoined, so it takes a quick moment to get used to the physical nuances of seeing the map on this extremity.

A Note on the Hairline

I am concerned with the original hairline when I assess and apply hands-on Reflexology to the face. Should the hairline be receded or not present, then I would use my visual assessment skills to determine where the hairline would have fallen. We could get into an entirely different discussion about the significance of a hairline being present, not being present and the timeline importance between those two states. Let's keep our focus strictly on the zones for now.

SAM BELYEA

FACE HORIZONTAL & VERTICAL ZONES

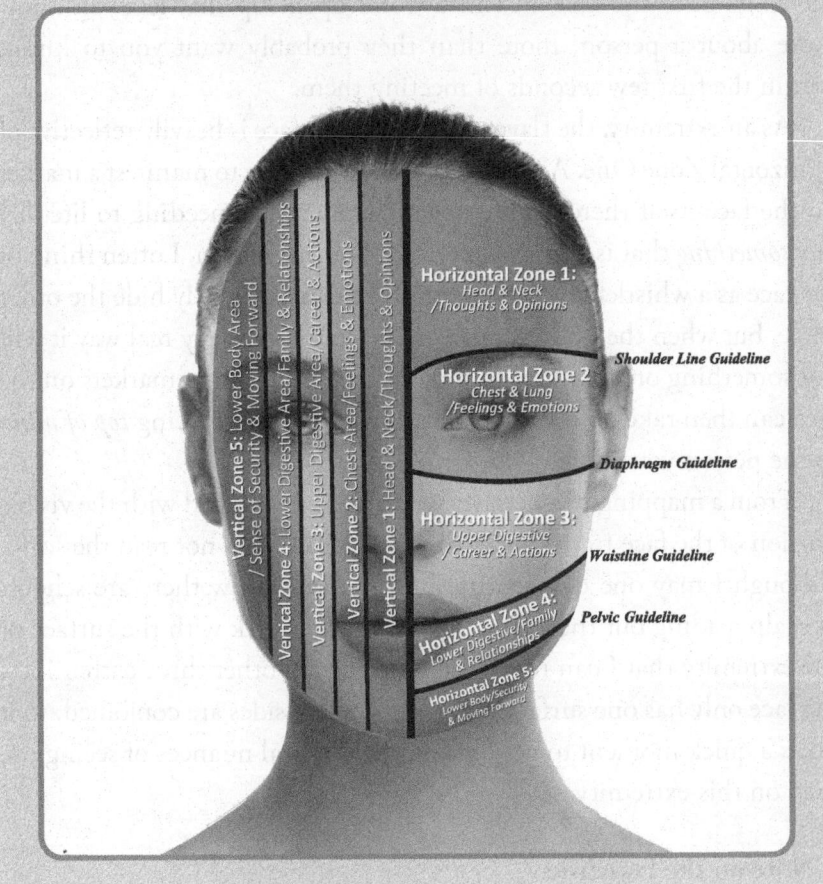

Horizontal Zone 1: Head & Neck /Thoughts & Opinions

Horizontal Zone 2: Chest & Lung /Feelings & Emotions

Horizontal Zone 3: Upper Digestive / Career & Actions

Horizontal Zone 4: Lower Digestive/Family & Relationships

Horizontal Zone 5: Lower Body/Security & Moving Forward

Shoulder Line Guideline
Diaphragm Guideline
Waistline Guideline
Pelvic Guideline

Vertical Zone 1: Head & Neck/Thoughts & Opinions
Vertical Zone 2: Chest Area/Feelings & Emotions
Vertical Zone 3: Upper Digestive Area/Career & Actions
Vertical Zone 4: Lower Digestive Area/Family & Relationships
Vertical Zone 5: Lower Body Area / Sense of Security & Moving Forward

Shoulderline Guideline:

The imaginary line that divides the head and neck structures from the chest, lung and shoulder area. Likewise, dividing the forehead of the face from the eyes by drawing a line at the eyebrows.

FOOT READING

Diaphragm Guideline:

The imaginary line that divides the chest, lung and shoulder area from the structures of the upper digestive system and upper core. Likewise, dividing the eyes from the upper cheeks by drawing a line along the Zygomatic ridge (*cheek bone*).

Waistline Guideline:

An imaginary line that divides the upper core from the structures of the lower core and pelvic area. Likewise, dividing the upper cheeks from the lower cheeks by continuing the natural line between the lips to extend to the lateral jaw.

Pelvic Guideline:

An imaginary line that divides the lower core and pelvic structures from the lower body. Likewise, dividing the lower cheeks from the jaw by drawing a line at the prominent base of the mandible (*jaw bone*).

Horizontal Zone One

<u>Location:</u> The Forehead
<u>Guideline:</u> Hairline & Shoulderline
<u>Physical Reflexes Present:</u> All structures of the head, neck and face. Including: Brain, Skull, Sinus, Eyes*, Teeth, Jaw, Ears*, Thyroid, Cervical Spine, Muscles/Bones of the Head and Face
<u>Mental/Emotional Meaning:</u> Thoughts and Opinions

To Reinforce: The forehead represents the structures head and neck. The neck in this case would be represented by the gentle curve above the eyebrows while the majority of the upper forehead would contain the reflexes for the actual head. I find the size of the forehead very significant to demonstrate the depth of the mind. If you notice in popular media, characters with intense mental capacity are framed with larger foreheads as a subconscious recognition of this zone's internal significance.

Horizontal Zone Two

Location: The Eyes
Guideline: Shoulderline & Diaphragm
Physical Reflexes Present: Shoulder, Lung, Heart (*more left side*), Ribs, Thymus, Breast, Arm*, Diaphragm (*technically on the Diaphragm Guideline*), Lymph Drainage, Upper Half of Thoracic Spine, Muscles/Bones of the Chest
Mental/Emotional Meaning: Feelings and Emotions

To Reinforce: The eyes are sometimes referred to as the window to the soul. I find the eyes to be more akin to the window into the heart when I do consultations. With the lateral temples representing the shoulder reflexes, and the innermost bridge of the nose representing the start of the thoracic spine, the eyes themselves represent the deep caves of the chest. So go the eyes, so goes the chest cavity. Be aware of left side eye issues because they represent activity in the heart reflex and present emotional tensions.

Left Eye Story: My partner Richard has a spontaneous left eye issue that began slowly and erupted into a real nasty mess – the same language could be used to describe the emotional situation surrounding the eye dysfunction. First, there was pain that slowly built into flashing light and a creeping black vein of color present in his field of vision. We were informed by an eye specialist that his retina had torn and was progressively detaching, which required an immediate cryo-surgery to prevent further disruption and heal the tear. All of this was terribly dramatic and traumatic for both of us, but the interesting details are in the background context while all of these markers were occurring.

Richard worked for a major company for fifteen years when word spread that there would be massive changes coming down the pipeline. After several turnovers in hierarchy and internal tensions mounting, Richard finally decided to leave the company to avoid even higher levels of stress. This all became clear as we took his blood pressure at our local grocery store, which turned out to be high – the first time he had high blood pressure in his life. Paired with the emotional stress pre-exit, it was no wonder that his left eye was the one incurring all the issues.

Upon leaving his job the eye no longer had pain or pressure, we measured his blood pressure again which had lowered well into normal levels and he had dropped about thirty physical pounds of stress related body fat. To this day I have not seen such a clear example of the reflexes at work than that left eye, blood pressure and current emotional situation.

Horizontal Zone Three

<u>Location:</u> The Upper Cheeks
<u>Guideline:</u> Diaphragm & Waistline
Physical Reflexes Present: Liver (*right*), Gallbladder (*right*), Pancreas (*more left*), Stomach (*left*), Spleen (*left*), Adrenal, Upper Half of Kidneys, Solar Plexus (*technically on Diaphragm Guideline*), Lower Half of Thoracic Spine, Muscles/Bones of the Upper Core
<u>Mental/Emotional Meaning:</u> Career and Actions

To Reinforce: When I work on faces, this zone presents terrible congestion on one side versus another. Little do clients know that stuffiness in their lower sinuses and issues in their upper teeth correspond to upper digestive and career distress. When assessing the face, you will largely be on the lookout for skin conditions such as Rosacea, Acne, superficial vesseling from excessive alcohol consumption and the occasional cold sore in this area of the face; each marker should be assessed individually. To refine your understanding of zones and structures, let me add that the right nostril relates to the Liver/Gallbladder duct reflex and the left nostril represents the esophagus reflex – depending on which nostril is clogged/draining will give you an idea of which upper digestive structure is complaining of discomfort.

Horizontal Zone Four

<u>Location:</u> The Lower Cheeks
<u>Guideline:</u> Waistline & Pelvic
<u>Physical Reflexes Present:</u> Large Intestine (*ascending and half of transverse on right; descending, sigmoid and half of transverse on left*), Small Intestine, Uterus/Prostate, Fallopian Tubes/Vas Deferens, Ovaries/Testes, Hip Joint (*TMJ*) Ureters, Bladder, Lower Half of Kidneys, Inguinal Lymph Drainage, Lumbar Spine, Muscles/Bones of the Lower Core
<u>Mental/Emotional Meaning:</u> Family and Relationships

To Reinforce: A fascinating change occurs when we see Horizontal Zone Four in hands and feet versus the face. The medial and lateral sides of the ankle and wrist represent the more medial and more lateral reproductive reflexes, but in the face, the reproductive reflexes are located more centrally at Horizontal Zone Four and Vertical Zones One & Two. The hip joint reflex is still laterally present in the masseter and TMJ area, along with the colon reflexes traversing the lower cheeks on either side, but the reproductive reflexes have shifted into the pocket of space between the jawline and the lower lip.

I first noticed this shift in the mapping on the face when several clients displayed beauty marks, moles, deep lines and skin conditions just over this small area of the face; the clients were all women having various stages of reproductive or hormonal distress. Likewise, when the face displays concentrated dysfunction within this area there is an ongoing theme of family/relationship stressors.

Horizontal Zone Five

<u>Location:</u> Jaw
<u>Guideline:</u> Pelvic
<u>Physical Reflexes Present:</u> Sciatic Nerve, Sacral Spine, Coccyx, Muscles/Bones of the Legs/Low Body
<u>Mental/Emotional Meaning:</u> Sense of Security and Moving Forward

To Reinforce: The lower prominence of the jaw represents everything in the lower body. This fact also connects frequent jaw pain with sciatic reflex issues on the side where they are present. The size of the jaw, or lack thereof, can give you a quick clue into how much energy the lower body has at its disposal. There can be a discrepancy between Horizontal Zone Five on the face being larger/smaller and Horizontal Zone Five on the feet being larger/smaller in comparison. I believe this discrepancy is caused by how stable and secure someone seems on the surface (*face*) versus how internally secure (*feet*) they feel about their life as a whole.

Vertical Zone One

<u>Location:</u> Midline of the Face to the Inner Corner of the Eye
<u>Physical Influences:</u> All reflexes found in Horizontal Zone One
<u>Mental/Emotional Influence:</u> Thoughts and Opinions

To Reinforce: The face doesn't have the neatly defined fingers and toes, but the Vertical Zones are still easy to find once you know what to look for. Instead of fingers and toes, I use the different sections of the eye to map the Vertical Zones starting with the space between the midline of the face and the inner corner of the eye to represent the influence of everything head and neck. Also, following this Vertical Zone down the face will help you understand the full extent of the spinal reflexes.

Vertical Zone Two

<u>Location:</u> The Inner Sclera of the Eye
<u>Physical Influences:</u> All reflexes found in Horizontal Zone Two
<u>Mental/Emotional Influence:</u> Feelings and Emotions

To Reinforce: Here I am mapping from the inner corner of the eye to the iris. This white section is known as the sclera, but what you will find very interesting is that this section of the eye will manifest specific markers when heavy feelings and emotions are occurring. Any marker in line with the inner sclera has that physical and internal influence of Horizontal Zone Two.

Vertical Zone Three

Location: The Iris of the Eye
Physical Influences: All reflexes found in Horizontal Zone Three
Mental/Emotional Influence: Career and Actions

To Reinforce: The colored lens of the eye and the pupil are both part of this Vertical Zone. The study of eyes known as iridology could be interjected here, but let's continue with just the basics. I find this Vertical Zone to be very helpful because it tells me that markers in line with the iris represent food-related conditions. Dietary issues are a quicker fix for those who are truly looking to make a difference. Some internal and physical combinations can occur in this zone when the person's work is preventing them from eating properly.

Vertical Zone Four

Location: The Outer Sclera of the Eye
Physical Influences: All reflexes found in Horizontal Zone Four
Mental/Emotional Influence: Family and Relationships

To Reinforce: When looking at someone in the eye, there is the inner white sclera of the eye and the outer white sclera of the eye. For Vertical Zone Four we are focused on that outer section. Everything in line with that section is being influenced by the physical and mental/emotional meaning of Horizontal Zone Four.

Vertical Zone Five

Location: Temples
Physical Influences: All reflexes found in Horizontal Zone Five
Mental/Emotional Influence: Sense of Security and Moving Forward

To Reinforce: Mapping the Vertical Zones of the face takes place in Horizontal Zone Two and moves from the midline of the face, across the eyes and finishes at the temples on either side of the eye complex. From the outside edge of the eye to outside edge of the face represents the Vertical Zone of Influence of Horizontal Zone Five's reflexes.

Mapping the Ears

Before I state my case for mapping the ears the way that I do, let me be sure to acknowledge that the Traditional Chinese Medicine (TCM) modality of Auricular Therapy is still very accurate – albeit the exact opposite of how I map the ears when I read them. How can I say that my way is different, but also affirm that the TCM method of ear manipulation and assessment is valid? Because I've seen both work splendidly. This book is not mean to criticize any one way of practice. Instead, I have written this text to inform you of the successes I have had; nothing more.

An Acupuncturist friend of mine and I would play a game within our networking group. When one of us saw the other assessing someone, the other would politely ask to 'grab an ear' and the game would begin. Both of us would be visually and texturally scouring the surfaces of the ear for information on what was causing this imbalance in the victim; who at this point was rather confused at the heated vigor with which we peered into their listening mechanisms – sometimes we would even draw a small crowd. The game would end as each of us stood back, side-stepped to discuss our findings.

To our utter amazement, we would come up with the exact same list of symptomology and root cause. The only difference was our language of choice to describe what we found and our methods for arriving at our conclusions. Other than that, we both would nail it! When you find someone who is good at what they do, regardless of the technique or training, you will get the same desired result. The same is true for mapping the extremities, but especially the ears in this case. I would get a little more insistent in regards to mapping the feet using Reflexology theory as a baseline, but that's back to my point of the feet being my extremity of choice.

An interesting observation I have made about the ears relates to the circumstances under which they manifest markers independently of the other three extremities. The flavor of the ears seems to be linked to its function in regards to hearing and listening. I have observed that the ears manifest markers relating to the soundtrack of our lives and issues that are specifically vocalized to us that the ears are responsible for intercepting. As an example, if you were told by a parent at an early age to choose a profession you hated and there was enough mental charge (*the ears are also heavily influenced by Horizontal Zone One*) to the situation, then a marker would warp the ear until the verbal assault on your nervous system was dealt with.

We hear words all the time, not every phrase or statement gets held onto by the body. I have just witnessed that when words are particularly striking to an individual, the timeline will match with a marker on the ear.

EAR HORIZONTAL & VERTICAL ZONES

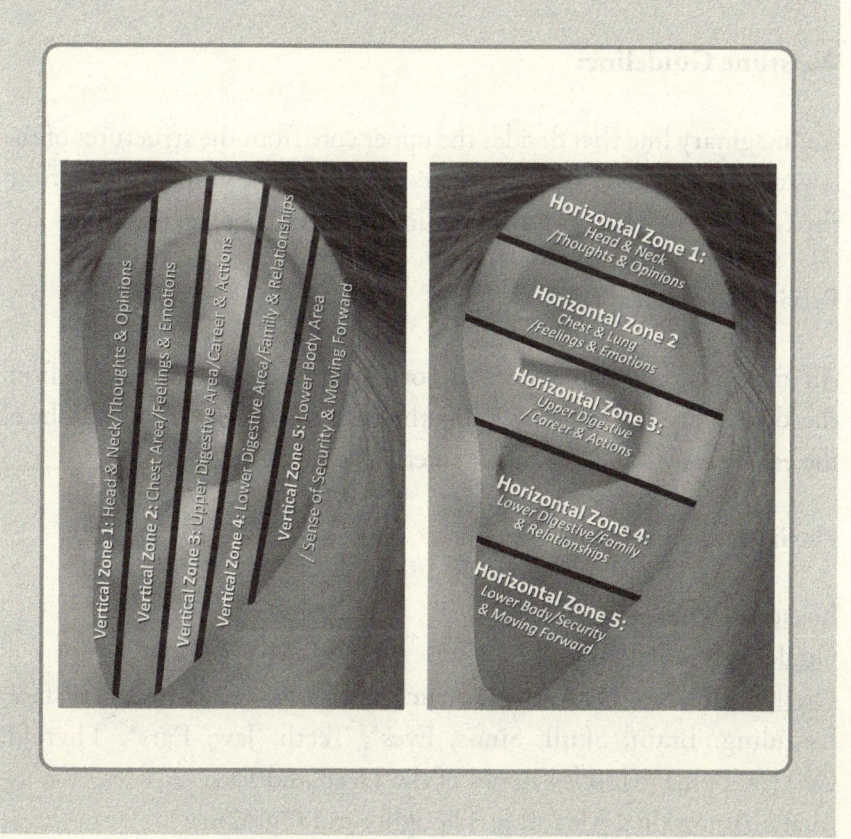

Vertical Zone 1: Head & Neck/Thoughts & Opinions
Vertical Zone 2: Chest Area/Feelings & Emotions
Vertical Zone 3: Upper Digestive Area/Career & Actions
Vertical Zone 4: Lower Digestive Area/Family & Relationships
Vertical Zone 5: Lower Body Area/Sense of Security & Moving Forward

Horizontal Zone 1: Head & Neck/Thoughts & Opinions
Horizontal Zone 2: Chest & Lung/Feelings & Emotions
Horizontal Zone 3: Upper Digestive/Career & Actions
Horizontal Zone 4: Lower Digestive/Family & Relationships
Horizontal Zone 5: Lower Body/Security & Moving Forward

Shoulderline Guideline:

The imaginary line that divides the head and neck structures from the chest, lung and shoulder area. Likewise, dividing the helix or top of the ear from the triangular fossa indentation by drawing a line at the eyebrows.

Diaphragm Guideline:

The imaginary line that divides the chest, lung and shoulder area from the structures of the upper digestive system and upper core. Likewise, dividing the triangular fossa indentation from the Cymba Concha or upper cave of the ear by drawing a line at the inferior crus of the antihelix.

Waistline Guideline:

An imaginary line that divides the upper core from the structures of the lower core and pelvic area. Likewise, dividing the Cymba Concha from the Cavum Concha by drawing a line at the crus of the helix.

Pelvic Guideline:

An imaginary line that divides the lower core and pelvic structures from the lower body. Likewise, dividing the Cavum Concha from the lobe of the ear by drawing a line at the intertragic notch.

Horizontal Zone One

Location: The Crest of the Helix
Guideline: Shoulderline
Physical Reflexes Present: All structures of the head, neck and face. Including: Brain, Skull, Sinus, Eyes*, Teeth, Jaw, Ears*, Thyroid, Cervical Spine, Muscles/Bones of the Head and Face
Mental/Emotional Meaning: Thoughts and Opinions

To Reinforce: The top of the ear represents the top of the body, just like with the other three extremities. Many people have interesting Horizontal Zone One shapes. Knowing your Vertical Zones is extremely important here. Remember that this zone within all the extremities represents the mental space of a person. The information collected from this zone can be very telling about how the imposed thoughts and feelings of others have shaped the framework of the person's mind.

FOOT READING

Horizontal Zone Two

<u>Location:</u> The Eyes
<u>Guideline:</u> Shoulderline & Diaphragm
<u>Physical Reflexes Present:</u> Shoulder, Lung, Heart (*more left side*), Ribs, Thymus, Breast, Arm*, Diaphragm (*technically on the Diaphragm Guideline*), Lymph Drainage, Upper Half of Thoracic Spine, Muscles/Bones of the Chest
<u>Mental/Emotional Meaning:</u> Feelings and Emotions

To Reinforce: This zone is technically present between the edges of the triangular fossa of the ear, which is the indent that rests between the crura of the antihelix. Lots of ear anatomy for you to look up in the section – I know I had to when I first started mapping the ear, but the purpose is so you know exactly where I am referencing in relation to specific zones. Capping off the zone in Vertical Zone Five is what is commonly referred to as Darwin's Tubercle. This may or may not be pronounced in the ear you are looking at, but the meaning is the same: the shoulder reflex.

A common marker I see in this zone is the presence of lightning in the ears. I call the marker that because there are raised colorful blood vessels that surface in this zone under severe emotional distress and chest/lung infections. It is something fun to look out for, but diligently note that the triangular fossa within this zone represents everything in the chest cavity.

Horizontal Zone Three

<u>Location:</u> The Cymba Concha
<u>Guideline:</u> Diaphragm & Waistline
Physical Reflexes Present: Liver (*right ear*), Gallbladder (*right ear*), Pancreas (*more left ear*), Stomach (*left ear*), Spleen (*left ear*), Adrenal, Upper Half of Kidneys, Solar Plexus (*technically on Diaphragm Guideline*), Lower Half of Thoracic Spine, Muscles/Bones of the Upper Core
<u>Mental/Emotional Meaning:</u> Career and Actions

To Reinforce: Similar to how the triangular fossa's indentation represents the chest cavity, so too does the indentation of the Cymba Concha represent the cavity of the upper core; housing all of the upper digestive organs on that particular side. However, the more lateral ridge of the outer ear does contain the more lateral structures which may include the tail end of the more lateral reflexes.

Horizontal Zone Four

Location: The Cavum Concha
Guideline: Waistline & Pelvic
Physical Reflexes Present: Large Intestine (*ascending and half of transverse on right; descending, sigmoid and half of transverse on left*), Small Intestine, Uterus/Prostate, Fallopian Tubes/Vas Deferens, Ovaries/Testes, Hip Joint (*TMJ*) Ureters, Bladder, Lower Half of Kidneys, Inguinal Lymph Drainage, Lumbar Spine, Muscles/Bones of the Lower Core
Mental/Emotional Meaning: Family and Relationships

To Reinforce: When clients refer to the ear, they often think of this part of the structure. The auditory opening leads into the inner ear, which we are not concerned with assessing. I will not shine a light into the ear and assess the canal, but I will take a peek around the auditory opening to survey for markers. This opening is a very active part of the ear and symptomology here can be diverse. The reflexes of the deep pelvis, reproductive, urinary and lower digestive structures all reside in this zone.

When surveying the ear, it is important to remember that the reflexes are through and through and that the back of the ear represents the back of the body. For this reason, the back of Horizontal Zone Four in the ear represents the lower back and glute area. Seeing the auditory opening as the deeper pelvic cavity is only part of the equation. Keep your eyes sharp for the multitude of surfaces within this zone!

FOOT READING

Horizontal Zone Five

<u>Location:</u> Lobe
<u>Guideline:</u> Pelvic
<u>Physical Reflexes Present:</u> Sciatic Nerve, Sacral Spine, Coccyx, Muscles/Bones of the Legs/Low Body
<u>Mental/Emotional Meaning:</u> Sense of Security and Moving Forward

To Reinforce: The lobe is the easiest part of the ear to assess with no frills or ridges. Lobe shape varies greatly from person to person. Most of my students believe that all ears are similar (*just like with the other three extremities*), but the lobe is an easy identifiable differentiation point that speaks to the nature of one's foundation. The flavor of this zone in the ear relies heavily on the dialogue surrounding their sense of security and moving forward, plus their thoughts about that process.

Whether a lobe is 'attached' or dangling does not matter as much as the overall size of this zone. The more/less tissue is present, the more/less physical and energetic weight is given to that zone. Assessing the lobes of the ears gives an easy contrast between sides of the body as well. Frequently there is a difference between the lobes from left to right and the meaning behind that alone could be the key factor that moves the needle for a consultation client.

Vertical Zone One

<u>Location:</u> From the Ear Attachment to the edge of the Tragus
<u>Physical Influences:</u> All reflexes found in Horizontal Zone One
<u>Mental/Emotional Influence:</u> Thoughts and Opinions

To Reinforce: More ear anatomy and it just keeps coming from here on in, so get out your anatomy books and pull up a search engine. The tragus is the flap that, if pressed in, would cover the auditory opening. When I refer to Vertical Zone One, I mean the curvy meandering tissue where the ear inserts to the head up until the edge of the tragus. This would also represent the spinal reflexes of the ear just as in Vertical

Zone One on the other three extremities. See? You just have to master the general layout and everything else falls into place!

Vertical Zone Two

Location: From Tragus to Antitragus
Physical Influences: All reflexes found in Horizontal Zone Two
Mental/Emotional Influence: Feelings and Emotions

To Reinforce: If you haven't pulled up that search engine by now, you're either really good at ear anatomy or you're going to shoot this book – so look it up! The antitragus is the flap of skin that looks like the tragus, but it sitting directly opposite the tragus in Horizontal Zone Four. This gap between the tragus and antitragus makes Vertical Zone Two and is also referred to as the intertragic notch. Just like in the other extremities, any marker that appears within this zone has heavy emotional and chest / lung / heart / shoulder reflex influence.

Vertical Zone Three

Location: The Antitragus
Physical Influences: All reflexes found in Horizontal Zone Three
Mental/Emotional Influence: Career and Actions

To Reinforce: Vertical Zone Three spans the width of the antitragus, so get familiar with this little hill. Markers in line with this anatomical landmark are associated with upper digestive influence; an influence that will differ depending on which ear the marker is on. Make sure you understand basic organ anatomy to get a better grip on the reflexes present and their influencing vertical zones for more specific interpretations.

Vertical Zone Four

<u>Location:</u> The Antihelix
<u>Physical Influences:</u> All reflexes found in Horizontal Zone Four
<u>Mental/Emotional Influence:</u> Family and Relationships

To Reinforce: Between the vertical space of the antitragus and the outer lateral edge of the helix is the ridge of the antihelix. When assessing the ear, you can easily identify this level as the second or middle step; with the first or lower step being the cavities of the ear and the third or higher step being the curled ridge of the helix that curls around the outer ear. The antihelix provides you with guidance on the influences of family and relationship dynamics as well as all of the Horizontal Zone Four reflexes, which can be numerous and sensitive.

Vertical Zone Five

<u>Location:</u> The Helix
<u>Physical Influences:</u> All reflexes found in Horizontal Zone Five
<u>Mental/Emotional Influence:</u> Sense of Security and Moving Forward

To Reinforce: Curving around the outside of the ear is the ridge known as the helix, which we use the crest of to mark Horizontal Zone One. This outer lip of the ear represents consistencies or inconsistencies with the lower body space and how that body section is influencing the other zones. This is a very interesting part of the ear to pay attention to and can be very dynamic in size and shape differences compared to the other zones. Really take note of how this zone compares to other ears you've seen and how someone's internal influence of moving forward corresponds.

Section Recap

- Although the feet are the focus of this text, the other extremities that can be mapped in the same way include the **Hands, Face and Ears.**
- Just like with the feet, we map the other three extremities with **Five Horizontal Zones and Five Vertical Zones.**
- There is **a general flavor to each extremity** that is highly influenced by the zone in which it is located, along with its form and function in the body.
- Some Foot Reading practitioners may find that they **resonate with a particular extremity** that may or may not include the feet.

The Story Continues with You

I mentioned at the beginning of this book that I feel this content is alive. This book is simply a manifested form of those living ideas; ideas that are shared across time and space with the rest of humanity who subconsciously have access to this same cluster of information. My final note to you in this book is to give you the ideas presented in this text and for you to run with them, letting the knowledge that has grown through me to continue its journey on through you so that its relevance can be spread to better serve the ecosystem of humanity. For you to do that, I am officially giving you a permission slip.

Note, I am not certifying you through these pages and no one can be an expert through reading a book. But, I challenge you to sop up the material contained within this book and let it come to life within your daily work. Whether you are a bodyworker, a home-based parent, an astronaut or a teacher, there is some unique way that this content can enrich your life and the lives of those around you. I ask for you to actively seek out that unique way and to let this living content flow into you as it has through me. Let the amazing and infinite intelligence present with the body to constantly wow you.

As I sit here, writing this closing chapter to a book that I feel marks the only beginning of my journey, I am filled with a sense of unending gratitude for the feet. I was someone who felt that the feet were just another part of a bigger body and had little meaning other than the fact that they were the ending part of a massage routine. Not knowing what I would learn. Searching for how it was all connected, but not finding the words or modality to accurately describe that connection.

The feet and indeed all four extremities are worlds of their own – divine in their own rite.

There is never a dull moment when you allow the magic of Foot Reading to share with you the mysteries hidden within yourself, another person or the makeup of our collective existence. I know that there is a lot of information in this book, but I encourage you to let the work work on you as much as possible. So, set this book down after you are done reading it and fall down the rabbit hole, as I did. Maybe our paths will cross someday and you will be able to share with me the amazing stories and experiences you have gained through reading the extremities.

Should you feel so called to work more on this topic and delve deeper into the content I have outlined in this book then please reach out to sam@footwhisperer.com so we can correspond. I also have Foot Reading videos on our YouTube channel, a Foot Reading & Reflexology Online Community (FRROC) group on Facebook and loads of extremity reading examples on our Instagram page (@footwhisperersam). Live and online classes are always popping up and can be accessed through www.footwhisperer.com, along with the ability to purchase our Foot, Hand, Face and Ear Reflexology charts. Believe me, this won't be my last book either so stay tuned for more works coming down the stream.

For now, go and get to work. There are a lot of feet out there waiting to be read by you and no one else can do it like you can. Happy travels and may the feet be with you (*I know, that was bad, but I had to do it*). Ciao!

Printed in the United States
By Bookmasters